Presenting in Biomedicine

500 tips for su   ss

Jane Fraser

and

Richard Cave

Radcliffe Medical Press

Oxford • San Francisco

Radcliffe Medical Press Ltd
18 Marcham Road
Abingdon
Oxon OX14 1AA
United Kingdom

www.radcliffe-oxford.com
The Radcliffe Medical Press electronic catalogue and online ordering facility. Direct sales to anywhere in the world.

British Library Cataloguing in Publication Data

A catalogue record for this book is available from the British Library.

ISBN 1 85775 897 8

Typeset by Advance Typesetting Ltd, Oxon
Printed and bound by TJ International Ltd, Padstow, Cornwall

Contents

About the authors

Dr Jane Fraser started her career as a research scientist, and has worked for more than two decades in biomedical publishing. She previously served as editorial director for two international medical communications agencies, during which time she developed many educational slide packages and helped researchers and physicians from around the world to put together more polished conference presentations. Since 1991, she has run her own company, providing training in scientific communications skills to universities, publishers and the pharmaceutical industry. She is a consulting tutor to the University of Oxford's Continuing Professional Development Centre and is the author of two previous books: *Professional Proposal Writing* (Gower, 1995) and *Publishing in Biomedicine: 500 tips for success* (Radcliffe Medical Press, 1997).

Dr Richard Cave has a PhD in organic chemistry and over 20 years' experience in the pharmaceutical industry. He has worked both internationally and at local company level, having held a number of senior sales and marketing positions in UK subsidiaries of two blue-chip pharmaceutical companies as well as gaining valuable experience in running a medical communications agency. Richard has a passion for developing people, which has characterised his management style. He now works as a management coach and trainer and has a particular interest in neurolinguistic programming, having qualified as a master practitioner. In addition he is a faculty member of the Chartered Institute of Marketing and of Management Centre Europe, and an associate lecturer at the University of Oxford.

Acknowledgements

The book grew out of the courses we each run in scientific communication, especially the Biomedical Presentations Skills Course we jointly teach as part of the University of Oxford's Continuing Professional Development Programme.

We would like to thank the many pharmaceutical and publishing companies, and the academic institutions that have commissioned courses over the years. Our gratitude is also due to the countless course participants, friends and colleagues who have contributed to our store of tips. Without them, this book could not have been written.

Jane Fraser
Richard Cave

Introduction

According to surveys (or is it a modern myth?), when people are asked 'what is your greatest fear?', speaking in public ranks second only to being burned alive. Even if your feelings about standing up to give a presentation are not quite as anguished as this, the fact that you're reading this book suggests that you are aware of the importance of good presentation skills in science.

For most biomedical researchers and academics, scientific presentations are an important part of their professional life. If you give conference talks or seminars, your presentation skills will determine how you – and your research – are perceived by your peers, superiors, and potential employers or grant awarding bodies. If you teach students, a good presentation will inform and inspire them, but a poor presentation will confuse and demotivate them.

Scientific presentations have come a long way since either of the authors was a student – at least in terms of technology. We now have presentation programs such as PowerPoint® to help us prepare professional-looking slides with the minimum of effort. We have digital technology that makes it easy to incorporate photography, video and sound into our presentations.

Much as we may enjoy these tools, however, we should bear in mind that scientists are by nature sceptics, and a flashy presentation cannot conceal dubious data. Moreover, technology can never compensate for your personal passion for your subject and your ability to communicate that knowledge and enthusiasm to your audience. Otherwise, you might as well email your presentation to the conference organisers and spend your time sightseeing instead.

Some people are 'natural' speakers, but it is not necessary to be an extrovert or an actor to be able to give a good presentation. We believe that, with good preparation and practice, *all* scientists can give competent, memorable presentations that will enhance their professional reputations. This book is designed to help you do just that.

Presenting need not be an ordeal. Contrary to what you might imagine in your darkest moments, your audience are willing you to succeed – they don't want to sit through a poor presentation any more than you want to give one.

We recognise that presenters have varying needs and different strengths and weaknesses, so this book is designed for you to use when you are actually preparing a presentation. It is intended to answer the commonest questions about scientific presentations, and to help you avoid the most common problems and pitfalls. You do not have to read it straight through from beginning to end – just dip into any chapter and you will find a range of tips relevant to the presentation you are preparing right now.

We hope that everyone who reads this book will find useful hints that they can use again and again, to help make preparing presentations easier, giving them more comfortable, and listening to them more pleasurable. Good luck, and we hope to see you on the podium!

For further information on courses on scientific presentation skills, contact:

Tailor-made courses for your organisation: Jane Fraser: www.janefraser.com; jane@janefraser.com; tel: +44 (0)161 9286684, or Richard Cave: www.members.trainerbase.co.uk/MorpheusLearning/; richard@morpheuslearning.co.uk; tel: +44 (0)1270 767486.

Open courses: Oxford University Continuing Professional Development Centre: www.conted.ox.ac.uk; anne.sheddick@conted.ox.ac.uk; tel: +44 (0)1865 286937.

1

Being invited to speak

It is always pleasant to be asked to give a presentation, and you may be so delighted and flattered that you accept immediately, no questions asked. But few things are more disconcerting than turning up at a meeting to discover that you are not speaking to the type of audience you had expected, or that the presentations of other speakers overlap substantially with yours.

▲ Don't be afraid to ask questions

Asking the right questions can help to ensure that you both you and your hosts are satisfied with your presentation. You will be much better prepared to give your presentation if you know a little about the reasons you have been invited to speak, the environment you will be speaking in, and what is expected of you.

▲ Is your brief obvious?

Often, you will have submitted an abstract to an organising committee, with the objective of presenting your own original research as an oral presentation or poster. Oral presentation is normally considered more prestigious, so if you receive an invitation to speak, you will be delighted. The subject matter will be obvious – you just go ahead and describe the study covered in your abstract. However, you will still need to find out some of the other information outlined below.

▲ Or does the subject matter need clarification?

If you are invited to speak at a plenary session giving a review of a particular topic, you may need to ask for more information. Has your presentation already been given a title, and if so what is it? Or are you required to submit a title to the organisers? If you have already been given a very broad title, you may need to probe further into which topics you are expected to cover, and the 'angle' from which you should approach them.

▲ Is there any flexibility in the choice of topic?

Occasionally, you may be asked to speak on something that you may not feel is really your area. Obviously, you could simply refuse the invitation. However, it may sometimes be possible to suggest a change to the title of your talk. Or, at the discretion of the meeting's organisers, it may be possible to 'swap' your topic with that of another speaker.

▲ Why have you been invited to speak?

If you are a Nobel Prize winner, the reason you have been chosen may be obvious. However, if the invitation comes 'out of the blue', it never does any harm to ask 'why me?' You may have published some recent interesting research in the field. Or perhaps someone in the audience at your last presentation was impressed with your performance and inspired to invite you to their meeting. Perhaps you are known (or assumed) to hold a particular point of view that either fits in with the spirit of the meeting, or is in opposition to that of another speaker. By asking 'why me?', you may gain information that will help you to meet your hosts' expectations more successfully.

▲ Who are your audience?

Sometimes the interests and information needs of your audience will be obvious. For example, if you are presenting to the members of a learned society, of which you are a member, you will already know a great deal about the kind of people who will be in the audience. On other occasions, you may not be so familiar with your audience – for example, if you are presenting your fundamental research on genetics to an audience comprised primarily of clinicians, you may need to find out a little about their interests and information needs before you begin to plan your talk.

Try this audience checklist

Some helpful questions to ask about your audience include:

- Who are they?
- What do they already know?
- What background information do they need to understand your talk?
- What interests them?

- What topics do they find irresistible?
- What turns them off?
- What technical vocabulary do they use?

▲ Who is chairing the meeting?

The chairperson is in charge of the scientific content of the meeting, and should be accorded appropriate respect. Usually, but not always, it will be the chairperson who actually telephones or writes to invite you to speak. If the invitation is made by someone else (e.g. the organising committee), it is useful to find out who *is* chairing the meeting – their name, address, phone, fax and email details – so that you can contact them if necessary. This is especially important if you are giving a review presentation, rather than simply talking about a particular study as specified in an abstract.

▲ Who else is on the programme?

If you are giving a review presentation, rather than simply speaking about your own research, it is well worth finding out who the other speakers are, the titles of their talks, and the order in which the presentations are to be given. This will enable you to prepare your talk to complement the presentations of the other speakers. If you are concerned about possible overlap, it may be necessary to talk to the other speakers to find out what topics they will be covering. It is most polite to do this via the chairperson, who may well have an opinion on which speaker should cover a particular topic.

▲ What is the date and time of your talk?

It may seem obvious, but you need to make a careful note of the date and time of your talk, and think about the practical implications for travel and accommodation arrangements. For example, if you are presenting first thing in the morning you will need to arrive the night before. Are you (or your institution) expected to fund your own travel and accommodation, or will your hosts or a sponsor pay your expenses? Who will actually make the arrangements? There may also be more subtle issues to be considered. If yours is the first talk of the day, it may fall to you to cover certain basic concepts central to the whole programme. If it is the first talk after lunch, you may need to think of ways in which to keep your audience interested and awake!

▲ Where is your talk being given?

Naturally, you need to know where you are going! You may need to check practical arrangements, such as getting a visa or immunisations for certain countries.

▲ Are there any cultural considerations?

In addition to practical matters, there may be cultural considerations in some countries. Are there any cultural references that would be inappropriate? Are there certain dress codes that apply in particular countries? If you plan to include a particular funny story in your talk, will it be understood, and is it likely to offend anyone? For example, references to visiting the bar may be innocuous enough in Europe or North America, but may not go down too well in countries where drinking alcohol is frowned upon.

▲ Can you work the country or city into your talk?

You may want to make an appropriate, flattering reference to the country or city in the content of your talk. For example, who were the early pioneers in your specialist subject in that country? Can you show a slide of their portrait, or the institution they worked in?

▲ How long should your talk last?

If it is not made clear in the invitation, you need to check how long your talk should last and how much time (if any) is to be allowed for questions.

▲ What about question time?

Check whether time will be allowed after each talk for questions, or whether questions will be taken at the end of each session.

▲ Will you be required to take part in a panel discussion?

In addition to answering questions on your own talk, you may be required to participate in a more general panel discussion. It is as well to be mentally prepared for this rather than to be surprised by it when you get to the meeting.

▲ How big will the audience be?

The size of the audience will influence the style of your talk. For example, if you are speaking to an audience of several hundred people at a major international congress, you will normally give your talk and take questions afterwards. The chairperson will determine which questioner should go next, and when the discussion should end. On the other hand, you may find yourself speaking at a more informal session, perhaps involving only a couple of dozen participants. In that case, there will probably be much more interaction, and you may decide to take questions as you go along. If the size and style of the meeting is not obvious, never be afraid to ask.

▲ Will you be using slides or the overhead projector?

Before preparing your presentation, you will need to know what audiovisual facilities will be available. Nowadays, it is standard practice to use Microsoft PowerPoint® or 35 mm slides for all major meetings. However, for small informal meetings and teaching sessions, overhead projection using acetates or a liquid crystal display (LCD) tablet is very acceptable (see Chapter 22).

▲ What slide projection facilities will be used?

If you plan to use slides, you will want to know:

- Are standard 35 mm slides to be used?
- Or will computer-projected PowerPoint slides be acceptable/compulsory?
- Will there be dual projection facilities?
- If so, will dual projection be used as standard or only if needed?

▲ Are you required to supply slide copy in advance?

Some meetings, usually those with a commercial sponsor, request speakers to provide slide copy in advance of the meeting. This is to enable the organisers to make all slides to a standard quality and format, or to prepare slides for computer projection (increasingly common). You may be delighted to have an opportunity to have your slides professionally prepared. On the other hand, you may prefer to use slides you already have in hand. So, if you are asked to provide slide copy, ask why it is wanted and whether it is compulsory or optional.

▲ What other audiovisual facilities will be available?

You may want to give a multimedia presentation, or show a video. You cannot automatically assume that the meeting will have the necessary facilities – it is important to enquire early about what is and is not possible. If showing a video is integral to your presentation, and the venue cannot provide the necessary facilities, it may be necessary to look into hiring them locally or even bringing them with you.

▲ Are you required to supply an abstract?

For an original research presentation, you will probably have already supplied an abstract to the organising committee, in order to get your contribution accepted. On the other hand, if you are an invited speaker, you may be asked to supply an abstract of your presentation. If so, don't forget to check:

- How long should the abstract be?
- Is it required as camera-ready copy on a standard form?
- If not, is it required in electronic format (e.g. by email)?

▲ Will there be a proceedings of the meeting?

It is important to know whether your presentation will be included in any proceedings of the meeting. If so, you will need to know the deadline for manuscript submission and have a copy of the relevant instructions to authors. Sometimes, your acceptance of an invitation to speak is deemed to indicate that you are willing to have a paper published in a proceedings. If your presentation includes original research, and you have submitted or are planning to submit a paper to another journal, there could be a potential conflict, as duplicate publication of original research is not allowed. If you have any doubts in this area, make a point of discussing the issues before you accept the invitation to speak.

2

Choosing your medium

We tend to think of talk-plus-slides as the natural medium for a scientific presentation, and it's true that this is often the most appropriate format. However, it isn't the only one. Even within the talk-plus-slides format, you will have some decisions to make. Here are a few tips to help you choose the best medium for your presentation.

▲ Choose your medium according to the presentation environment

There are many options available to help you get your message across to the audience. Which you select will depend on the location, the technology available, the type of meeting (i.e. degree of formality), the size of the audience and your past experience.

▲ You may not need any visual aids for an informal talk

If you have been invited to address a small group informally, you may not need visual aids – you yourself are the best visual aid. This format is suitable for impromptu presentations to small groups, e.g. a tutorial session, or a presentation at a selection interview.

▲ Even presentations to large audiences do not always require slides

Not all presentations by scientists or clinicians are full of scientific data. Some rely more on the passion and persuasiveness of the speaker. If you find yourself in such a situation – for example, presenting to schoolchildren on 'why I became a doctor' – consider whether you really need visual aids. One of the most powerful presenters I know is a welfare officer for a medical charity. When she has to present at international medical congresses, she often does so without notes or slides. Her talk thus appears to come straight 'from the heart', though in fact the content is carefully considered. Her personal, unashamedly emotional presentation provides a vivid contrast to the more 'scientific' presentations on the programme.

▲ In small, highly interactive groups, consider using a flipchart or blackboard

Drawing your visual aids as you go may seem old-fashioned, but it can sometimes be useful. For example, you might want to summarise participants' comments, or to develop a protocol or algorithm into which participants can provide input. 'Low-tech' methods such as pre-drawn flipcharts are also appropriate in any situation in which you feel you cannot rely on technology – for example, in remote locations. For tips on using flipcharts effectively, see Chapter 21.

▲ Overhead projector transparencies are still a useful 'low-tech' option …

Today, overhead projector (OHP) transparencies may seem a little old-fashioned compared with more high-tech presentation methods. Yet they are still extremely useful. Some small venues may not be able to offer a slide projector or data projector, but do have an OHP available. For tips on using OHP acetates effectively, see Chapter 22.

▲ … And are more flexible than standard 35 mm slide shows

Standard 35 mm slides, sitting in a pre-arranged order in their carousel, make it difficult to be flexible about the order in which you present your information. Computerised presentations, using PowerPoint or a similar program, are much more flexible, but the necessary facilities may not always be available. If you anticipate the need for flexibility in your presentation, moving backwards and forwards within your slides or leaving some out altogether, and you do not have access to a data projector, overhead transparencies may be your next best option.

▲ Standard 35 mm slides are still required at many conferences …

There is no doubt that 35 mm slides are gradually being superseded by computerised presentations. However, there are still some meetings where the conventional photographic film in glass mounts remains the preferred format. There is a good financial reason for this – many venues have yet to invest in the expensive data projectors needed to give a good quality image in a large conference hall. The downside of 35 mm slides is that their preparation is time-consuming and last-minute changes are impossible.

▲ ... But the computer-generated presentation is fast becoming the standard

Many scientists are now used to preparing their presentations using computer software, and delivering them using a computer and linked data projector (also known in some countries as a 'beamer'). The most popular program is PowerPoint, but others are also available. In the industrialised countries, computerised presentations are fast becoming the standard method – though no doubt the technology will continue to advance and change.

▲ Don't forget that you can present to small groups using a monitor or television (TV) screen

If you want to give a computerised presentation to a small group, you may not even need a data projector. If you are presenting to just two or three people, you can gather them round your laptop or a computer monitor. For slightly larger groups, you may be able to present via a TV screen.

▲ Be open to the new opportunities offered by computerised presentations

With computerised presentations, you are not restricted to simple slides, but can give multimedia presentations, incorporating (for example) animations, video clips and web pages – anything you can create or view on your computer, you can project on a screen with a data projector. The computer also makes it easier to go backwards and forwards in your presentation, and to amend and add material on the spot.

▲ Investigate exactly what technology will be available ...

Before you get carried away with creating your PowerPoint presentation, check exactly what technology you will be using. For example, will you be using the host institution's computer, or will you be bringing your own laptop? If you're using an unfamiliar computer, how powerful is it and what software is it running? There's no point in creating an all-singing, all-dancing multimedia presentation if you will end up trying to give it on a computer that can't cope. More tips on using PowerPoint and similar programs are given in Chapters 11–20.

▲ ... And who will operate it

Just because the venue has the facilities for computerised presentations doesn't mean that you will necessarily be controlling the presentation yourself from the lectern. Many venues do provide the speaker with a screen and keyboard on the lectern, so that they can control the computer themselves. However, at other meetings, presentations may be controlled by a professional operator, so that deviating from the pre-arranged order of slides becomes difficult or impossible.

▲ Don't forget that you can distribute computerised presentations on the Internet

Having created your computer-generated presentation, it is also possible to put it onto a website. It can then be made available to a much larger audience and downloaded if desired. Alternatively you may wish to email your presentation to your audience. Don't forget that very large files will need to be compressed ('zipped') to make transmission faster.

▲ Use video when it will add to your message

Video, whether as part of a multimedia presentation or inserted into a 'traditional' talk-and-slides presentation, is invaluable for demonstrating moving objects. For example, you might want to demonstrate a surgical procedure, or an animal, person or machine in motion. For more tips, see Chapter 23.

▲ Remember that you can use a data projector for more than just showing slides

The data projector can of course be used to demonstrate computer programs or show the content of an Internet or Intranet page, as well as to show slides. Be sure to test that everything works in advance of the presentation, as described below.

▲ Work on the principle that if technology can go wrong, it will

Nothing falls flatter than a presentation in which the technology doesn't work. Make sure that the equipment you are using works in the exact configuration you will be using on the day. It is worth going to some trouble to do this. If anything changes between setting up the equipment and actually giving the presentation, check it again. If you are relying on a modem connection to give a demonstration, check it repeatedly to ensure that it is dependable. If someone else is handling the techno-logical side of things, make sure they know your requirements.

▲ Don't forget the power of the 'live' demonstration ...

Sometimes a simple demonstration can be a very effective way of delivering your message. For example, in a clinical presentation, a short interview with a patient is much more memorable than a list of symptoms on a slide.

▲ ... And audience participation

Audience involvement can do a lot to add interest to your presentation. Questions are of course a form of audience involvement (for advice on handling questions, see Chapter 34). But there are other possibilities – you could ask for volunteers to help you in a demonstration, or simply conduct a show-of-hands survey of opinion or experiences. If asking for audience opinion is to be a major part of the presentation, it is even possible to use interactive keypad systems that will analyse responses to multiple-choice questions and show the results via computer software.

▲ Videoconferencing can be used to show a presentation or procedure to a remote audience

You may be asked to give a presentation that will be transmitted to a remote audience via videoconferencing facilities. Videoconferencing can also be used to transmit a practical demonstration, e.g. a surgical procedure. The style of presentation needed is quite didactic. You need to be very deliberate in your delivery, carefully describing what the audience is looking at. Although questions often form an important part of the videoconference presentation, these need to be presented formally one-by-one. Generally speaking, it is not possible to engage the audience to the same degree as in a face-to-face talk.

3

Researching your presentation

If you are presenting an original research study, the content of your talk will be obvious. However, if you are giving a presentation that includes any components of review, you may have to do some background research. This can be a little or a lot, depending on the presentation.

▲ Review what you already have

The first step is to review the information you already have. Often, this is done in parallel with preparing an outline for your talk (see Chapter 4). Remember to look not only at facts and supporting papers, but at potential slides.

▲ Keep your eyes open for interesting illustration ideas

One of the commonest problems in preparing presentations is a shortage of interesting illustrative material. Once you have reviewed your current store of information and illustrations, you will be able to identify gaps and set about filling them.

▲ Don't try to do it alone

If you are new to making presentations, you will feel a lot more confident if you prepare your presentation with the help of a suitably critical but sympathetic adviser. This could be your research supervisor or boss, or simply a more experienced colleague. Friends and partners can also be pressed into service to give an honest opinion of both the content and delivery of your presentation.

▲ Beg and borrow ...

If you don't have all the information you need, don't be shy about asking your colleagues for help. They may well have covered the same ground before, and be able to supply you with background materials and even slides for you to use in your presentation. Provided permission is given, borrowing is a useful short cut – why spend hours in the library if it's not necessary?

▲ ... But never steal

It's perfectly normal to make reference to the work of others, especially in review presentations. However it is important to keep track of exactly which study your information comes from, and to make due acknowledgement of the authors in your presentation. It is acceptable to show slides based on figures published by others, but the original source must always be acknowledged. If you use unpublished data in your talk, you must *always* obtain permission from the original source.

▲ Use online databases

Online searches, whether you conduct them yourself or have them done by an information specialist, can help you to be sure that you have not overlooked any relevant studies. This is important both for review presentations and for putting your own research into context.

▲ Think about questions as well as the talk itself

Knowledge of the relevant background will help you to be prepared for awkward questions. After all, some of the people who conducted studies that reached opposing conclusions may be in the audience, and all too ready to stand up for their opinions. If you pre-empt at least some of their comments by mentioning their studies, some of the heat may be taken out of the debate.

▲ Make sure you are up to date

It is important to be aware of the most recent research relevant to your talk. Online databases will be helpful here, but they may not give you information published in the last couple of weeks. Nor will they tell you about research presented at congresses, but not yet published. If you're talking about your own specialist field, you will probably have your finger on the pulse of research and of the latest developments from others in the field. If you're talking outside your normal area, or on a broad topic, you may need to ask colleagues closer to the action for the very latest information.

▲ Use the resources of the Internet

Get to know the relevant resources on the Internet – not only websites, but newsgroups. You can 'lurk' around the newsgroups without contributing to them, if you prefer. While there is a lot of irrelevant and 'oddball' material on the Internet, there is also a great deal that is useful – the trick is to identify the most authoritative sites. If you work in clinical medicine, the Internet provides a useful insight into the perspectives of patients and 'consumers' of healthcare – viewpoints that you might like to mention in your talk.

▲ Watch TV and read magazines

Science programmes on TV and magazines such as *New Scientist* and *Scientific American* are very adept at making science understandable and interesting, even for non-scientists. You can often pick up useful tips on how to present your own material to a scientific audience in a more interesting and enjoyable way.

▲ Keep a 'talks file'

Every time you come across something that could be useful in a future talk, photocopy it and file it in your 'talks file'. That way, when you're next asked to give a talk, you will already have a store of useful ideas at your fingertips.

4

Outlining your presentation

Very few of us can give a successful presentation without careful preparation. Most presenters, even the most experienced, like to prepare a detailed outline. Preparing such an outline will give you confidence that you have not missed any important topics when preparing your presentation. If you have your outline in front of you during your talk, it will also help you to keep on track, even if you become nervous or distracted.

▲ Begin from your conclusion

Every presentation has a conclusion, 'bottom line' or 'take-home message'. Ask yourself: 'After this presentation, what do I want my audience to:

- think?
- believe?
- decide?
- do?'

▲ In original research, your conclusion will be the answer to a question …

In original research, your conclusion is always the answer to the question posed at the beginning of the research. Every study sets out to answer a specific question, which follows logically from what is already known. If you don't know what question your research set out to answer, you are not ready to start preparing your presentation.

▲ ... Sometimes the question itself is the topic of the presentation

Sometimes you will have the opportunity to describe a study in progress. For example, you may be involved in a large, important trial for which no results are available as yet. In that case, the topics of your presentation will be the reasons for the study, the questions it is designed to answer, and the methods used.

▲ Make your conclusion powerful

You should be able to write your conclusion in one sentence. Positive statements with the minimum of 'ifs' and 'buts' usually make the most powerful conclusions. Very often, the 'bottom line' will form part of the introduction to your talk (see below). For example: 'This presentation describes our study showing that X is an effective treatment for Y in patients with Z'; 'Today I'm going to present what I believe to be the overwhelming evidence that ...'; 'This presentation will enable you to diagnose Heffenpfeffer's disease more accurately in your elderly patients'.

▲ Write your conclusion down and make sure everything you say is relevant to it

Planning a talk is a lot like planning a journey. Deciding on the route is much easier once you know your destination! Once you know your conclusion, you can marshal the facts you need to support it, and the logical order in which those facts and ideas should be presented. You can use various planning techniques to help you do this, described in the following tips. Which technique you choose is not important – you may well have tried and tested methods of your own. What *is* important is that you have a plan.

▲ Try mind mapping

Mind mapping is a technique popularised by psychologist Tony Buzan. It is based on the idea that people do not naturally think in rigid hierarchies or lists. Instead, the human mind darts around from subject to subject, moving naturally and creatively from one topic to another, 'growing' one idea from another. Mind mapping is a way of capturing this 'radiant thinking' in a visual form, which can then be used to develop a more rigid structure.

▲ Try the 'yellow sticky' note technique for organising ideas ...

Another way of making sense of a large number of ideas is to jot down key topics in note form on 'yellow sticky' Post-it® notes. You can then lay these out on your desk – or even the wall or floor – and move them round until an appropriate plan emerges. You can combine this technique very effectively with mind mapping (see above).

▲ ... And their associated references

Another way of using the 'yellow sticky' approach is to write one Post-it® note for each reference, noting the author and title of the reference and the key points you want to extract from it. You can then move these around as before – a great way of planning review presentations.

▲ Try building pyramids of ideas

A pyramid consists of a single brick at the top (the 'big idea' of the article). Under this are several bigger bricks (supporting facts or ideas), and under these more smaller bricks (smaller facts or ideas). Make sure that you introduce the big bricks first, before going on to support them with the smaller bricks. Never have piles of little bricks lying around with no discernible structure.

▲ Try using the outline function on your word processor

Most well-known word-processing programs, including Word and Word Perfect, have an outline function that will allow you to organise your ideas as a hierarchy of headings. An outline of this kind will help you to define your main sections, subsections and sub-subsections. However, it is often best to precede this phase of planning with a more open phase such as mind mapping, to make sure you don't get stuck in the rut of straight-line thinking.

▲ Set yourself a time budget

A time budget is a plan allocating a certain number of minutes to each section of the presentation. Setting such a budget will help you to:

• avoid wasting time researching ideas and graphics you will never have time to cover
• assign the right balance of material to each section.

▲ Be ruthless

You will hardly ever have time to say everything you want to say, so you will have to be ruthless at the planning stage. Otherwise you will find yourself having put together 50 slides for a ten-minute presentation, and having to decide which ones should be axed. For the sake of your time and your peace of mind, it's far better to get it right first time round.

▲ Plan slides and content in parallel ...

(The term slides is used here to cover 35 mm slides, OHP acetates and audiovisual materials.) Most experienced presenters find it easiest to plan slides and the spoken presentation that goes with them in parallel.

▲ ... Or start with the slides

If you already have an extensive range of slides prepared, you may be able to start by making a selection of slides, then prepare your talk around them. But be careful not to overlook any gaps in your logic that should be filled by preparing a new slide.

For more tips on planning research presentations, see Chapters 5–7.

5

Presentation structure: getting started

As in every other aspect of life, first impressions are vitally important. These tips will help you to get your presentation off to a good start.

▲ Make a good impression in the first 30 seconds

It's often said that the first 30 seconds of any person-to-person encounter create an indelible first impression, and that includes your first encounter with the audience for your presentation. If it's good, that first impression will carry you a long way, even if you run into trouble later on.

▲ Rehearse the opening repeatedly

If the first impression is bad, you will have to work doubly hard during the rest of the presentation to retain the audience's attention, interest and trust. So it pays to rehearse repeatedly to make sure your first impression is perfect. Consider all the aspects – not only the words you use, but the volume and tone of voice, body language, eye contact, and of course your personal appearance. You'll be nervous, so practise until standing up and saying your opening words becomes automatic.

▲ 'Tell them what you're going to tell them ...'

You've almost certainly heard the old advice on giving a presentation: 'Tell them what you're going to tell them, tell them, then tell them what you've just told them.' It's trite but true. Any effective talk requires a beginning, middle and end, and key messages need to be repeated at least three times to be absorbed.

▲ Spend time and trouble crafting your introduction

Your introduction sets the tone for the whole talk, so it's worth giving it considerable thought. A good introduction will provide the audience with the answers to the following questions:

- Who are you?
- What are you going to talk about?
- When are you going to stop?
- Where is it going?
- Why should I listen?
- How are you going to make it interesting?

▲ Write your introduction last

If you can't imagine how you will get started, put off thinking about it until you've finished putting together the rest of the talk. Often, you'll find the right beginning comes to you naturally when you've refined the messages in the body of the talk and the conclusions.

▲ Be polite, but don't waste too much time on elaborate greetings

It is usually appropriate to greet the audience and chairperson, but don't spend too much time on greetings. The polite way to start will depend on the country you're in – if in doubt, ask someone what would be the appropriate thing to say. In Europe and North America, 'Good morning, ladies and gentlemen, Professor Smith' is usually enough. Only attempt to greet audiences in a foreign language if you are quite sure you can do it correctly and confidently. You can skip the greetings altogether if you are talking to people you already know, e.g. in a departmental seminar.

▲ Limit the length of the introduction

People will be anxious to get to the meat of your talk, so don't spend too long on introductory material – especially if your talk is very short. As a rule of thumb, if you spend more than ten per cent of the total talk time introducing yourself and your topic, it's too long.

▲ Make sure the audience knows who you are …

Unless you are so well known you truly are one of those people who 'needs no introduction', you need to be sure that the audience knows who you are. Usually the chairperson will introduce you, but if not, then be sure to say something along the lines of 'Good morning, ladies and gentlemen. I'm Jane Doe of the Department of Nursing Studies at the University of Wherever, and today I'm going to be talking about …'

▲ … And what you're going to be talking about

The chairperson may have stated what you're going to be talking about, and it may also be in the programme, but it doesn't hurt to remind the audience what your topic is: '… and today I'm going to be talking about the role of the specialist nurse in the management of heart failure, and in particular our recent study on …'

▲ You might need to tell the audience how long your talk will last

Often, the audience will know from the programme that everyone will be giving talks of a certain length. But if, for any reason, this is not clear, make it your business to tell them: 'I plan to talk for about half an hour, and then we'll have 15 minutes for questions.' People relax and listen better if they know how long the talk will last, and they will certainly be in a better mood if they know when to expect coffee and lunch breaks.

▲ Give people a reason to listen early in the introduction

Early in your introduction, try to provide a subtle (or not so subtle) answer to the audience's unspoken question 'what's in it for me?'. Sometimes the answer is more or less obvious (e.g. information for people interested in the results of your research study). However, especially if your talk does not seem immediately relevant to this audience, it may be useful to slip in a motivating statement early on. For example, if you are a geneticist speaking to clinicians: 'I'm going to describe recent findings on the genetics of cystic fibrosis that may, in the future, have important implications for its clinical management.'

▲ The introduction can also offer the audience a preview of items of special interest

You can increase the audience's predisposition to listen by mentioning one or two highlights of your talk in the introduction. For example, 'In addition to reviewing the results of the THINGY study, I'll be presenting for the first time some new results from a subgroup analysis that show elderly patients respond just as well to thingacin as younger patients', or 'I'll be illustrating my talk with video clips showing the process taking place inside a live animal …'.

▲ In a research talk, give only necessary background

If you are speaking specifically about your own research, you should not attempt to give a comprehensive overview of the whole area before you start talking about your own study. You should aim to give only the background information needed to enable people to understand why you did the research. Your objective is not to educate the audience, but to prepare them to understand your research and put it into context.

▲ Check with other speakers to avoid overlap

If someone else is speaking on a similar topic, their introduction may overlap substantially with yours. Rather than wait until the day of the presentation to find out that they've 'stolen' all your best ideas, why not give them a call beforehand, so that neither of you looks foolish on the day.

▲ To focus the audience's mind on a new topic, try using one of these devices

In a very brief scientific presentation, you may have to plunge straight into the 'meat' of your talk. However, especially if your talk is on a different topic from previous presentations, you can use one of the devices detailed below to get the audience's attention and mentally move them on to a new topic.

Option 1: Anecdote

'I'd like to tell you about the first time I ever saw a case of Snodgrass syndrome.' Keep it short and make sure you show why it's relevant.

Option 2: Occasion

'I'm delighted to be able to contribute to this symposium honouring the retirement of Professor Snodgrass …'

Option 3: Importance

'Snodgrass syndrome is the third leading cause of death in most industrialised countries …'

Option 4: Refer to previous talks

'Dr Adams has just underlined the importance of obesity as a risk factor for Snodgrass syndrome. I'm going to focus my talk on a related risk factor: physical inactivity ...'

Option 5: Humour

You can begin with a relevant funny story, but you need to be sure:

- you can tell it with confidence and style
- the whole of the audience will understand and relate to it
- the audience has not heard it before
- no one in the audience will be offended by it
- none of the other speakers have used it.

Option 6: Example

'Here's the ECG of a patient seen recently in our clinic. It reveals the three cardinal features of Snodgrass syndrome ...'

Option 7: History

'In 1886, this man, William Snodgrass, was the first to describe a syndrome that continues to perplex scientists today ...'

Option 8: Definition

'According to *Stedman's Medical Dictionary*, Snodgrass syndrome is defined as ...'

Option 9: Fact or statistic

'This year, in North America alone, nearly 10 000 people will die from Snodgrass syndrome ...'

Option 10: Quote

'William Snodgrass called the syndrome named after him "one of the most fascinating and frustrating disorders known to man" ...'

Option 11: Question

'What are the key risk factors for Snodgrass syndrome, and how can we prevent it?'

Option 12: Reference to a place or institution

'I'm delighted to be talking about Snodgrass syndrome at the university where Snodgrass himself studied ...'

▲ Be sure that you understand the procedure for starting your slides

With computerised projections becoming the norm, it's important to think about how to achieve a smooth and professional transition into your presentation. It's irritating for the audience to have to watch lots of fussing about starting up programmes and finding files, and it eats into valuable presentation time. You might have to provide the organisers with a disk or CD before the sessions starts, to be loaded onto a single computer. You'll need to check whether someone will be switching to your slides at the appropriate moment, or whether you'll have to find the file yourself (if so, the easiest thing to do is to place a shortcut to it on the desktop).

▲ Ideally, the first thing the audience sees should be your introductory slide

With computerised presentations, it's most professional-looking if you can arrange for the screen to be blanked out while the change-over is made so that the first thing they see is an introductory slide. Sometimes, a slide with the logo of the conference or a relevant photo is shown while change-overs are made between presentations.

▲ Be ready to start as soon as the previous speaker has finished

It sounds obvious that you should have your notes and slides organised, and be ready to start as soon as the previous speaker has finished. But it's all too easy to get into a muddle, especially if the previous speaker finishes a little early or there are no questions after their talk. It's unsettling and irritating for the audience to watch you fussing around getting yourself ready.

▲ Don't apologise for your presentation

If you are feeling nervous about your presentation, you may be tempted to share your feelings with the audience by saying things like, 'Unfortunately I can't promise to be as interesting as the previous presentation ...'; 'Please bear with me as I take you through some rather difficult statistics ...'. Don't. You have as much right to be there as the previous speaker. If your presentation is truly boring, either decline the invitation or find a way of making it more interesting.

▲ Avoid running on autopilot

Most presentations will run according to plan. But there may be occasions when events overtake you. For example, despite all your efforts to plan and predict, a previous speaker may have covered some of the same ground as you. If circumstances change, do your best to respond, for example by missing out some of your slides and spending more time on others.

▲ Don't be a 'tourist'

It's acceptable to make reference to the country or city in which you're presenting, especially if you can highlight some aspect relevant to your talk. But don't let this lapse into a travelogue of your sightseeing tour of the city – stick to the point of your presentation.

6

Presentation structure: the body of the talk

Most of your presentation time will be devoted to the body of the talk – the part where you summarise your research or put forward your main arguments. Here are some tips to help you organise your talk at the detailed level.

▲ Remember that a research talk does not necessarily follow the same structure as a research paper

It's easy to assume that a research talk will follow exactly the same pattern as a research paper. It's true that they have many points in common – both will include an introduction, followed by information on the methods used, the results obtained, a discussion of those results, and some kind of conclusion or summing up. But a talk is not constrained by the rigid format of a scientific paper. You can use whatever structure you think will work best, remembering that you should try to maintain the audience's interest throughout the talk.

▲ For research presentations, use the standard format

For research presentations, it is usual to begin with an introduction, followed by the methods, results, discussion and conclusion – the same format as in scientific papers. In other words (to paraphrase Maeve O'Connor):[1]

- Why did you start?
- What question did you ask?
- What did you do?
- What did you find?
- What does it mean anyway?

▲ To structure a research talk, ask yourself three key questions

- Do you want to wake your audience up with some conclusions at the beginning, or would you prefer to save them all for the end?
- If several different methods were used, would it be more logical to give the relevant results following the description of each method (rather than giving all the methods followed by all the results, as often happens with scientific papers)?
- Do you want to discuss each individual result as soon as you present it? Or do you need to state all the results before you draw the different strands together at the end?

▲ Spend most of your time on what interests the audience most

One of the most important differences between a paper and a presentation is the balance between methods and the results. In a scientific paper, the methods often constitute the longest section because you have to give sufficient detail to allow the study to be repeated by others. This criterion is not applied to presentations. Unless your methods were particularly interesting or unusual, the audience is likely to be much more interested in your results, so it is both permissible and advisable for your results to take up much of your presentation time.

▲ Don't dwell on the negative aspects of your study

In the discussion section of a scientific paper, you're required to discuss any limitations of your study, conflicts between your results and those of other researchers, or inconsistencies within your own results. You may mention these in your talk, but don't dwell on them or you risk ending up with a negative impression. Remember that you can always address any contentious issues during question time – and if the audience doesn't draw attention to a problem, why should you?

▲ For reviews, try one of these standard approaches

Every review presentation is different, but listed below are a few general approaches that can be used for a variety of subjects. You can of course combine several different types of approach in one talk.

Option 1: Historical

You might include past research, present knowledge and the next steps.

Option 2: Problem-solving

State the problem, offer proposed solutions with advantages and disadvantages, and conclude with the preferred solution.

Option 3: Inductive reasoning

State the research question, offer evidence and end with logical conclusions.

Option 4: Comprehensive

Tell the audience everything they always wanted to know about headlice but were afraid to ask.

Option 5: Selective

Stick to a strictly limited brief, e.g. five essential rules for managing headlice.

Option 5: Personal

Look at the problem from your own or someone else's point of view, e.g. one family's experience of headlice.

Option 6: Comparative

Compare and contrast between approaches to a problem, e.g. healthcare systems in one country versus another.

Option 6: Metaphorical

Occasionally, a sustained metaphor may bring your subject alive. Real-life examples where we've seen this approach work well include heart failure as a maze through which the cardiologist must find a route, and the search for a cure for Parkinson's disease as a search for the Holy Grail.

▲ Construct 'bridges' from one part of your talk to another

When you move on to a new topic, use 'bridging' devices to help the audience to follow the flow. Examples include:

- **previews** – 'I'll be describing this in more detail later'
- **interim summaries** – 'So, let's review where we were this time last year in terms of our knowledge of such-and-such'.

The longer the talk, the more of these bridges you need.

▲ Use 'attention grabbers' to help the audience stay alert

Audiences cannot maintain the same level of attention over a long period, so use specific things to help focus attention on key points. Typical attention grabbers might include:

- arresting visuals
- case histories
- anecdotes
- quotations
- startling statistics
- analogies
- practical points to remember.

▲ Think of your presentation like an action movie

If you've ever watched an action movie like the 'James Bond' series, you'll know that it's punctuated by exciting moments at regular intervals. Unlike a scientific paper, in which most of the exciting material is found relatively near the end, your talk should have interesting material throughout in order to hold the audience's attention. Like an action movie, it should begin in an exciting way and end in a grand finale that ties up all the loose ends.

▲ Reference

1 O'Connor M (1991) *Writing Successfully in Science*. Chapman and Hall, London.

7

Presentation structure: classy conclusions

Every presentation should have a conclusion. People tend to remember the last things that they see and hear, so make sure your conclusion is powerful, memorable and well-rehearsed.

▲ Always have a conclusion

It's satisfying to the audience to have the presentation nicely rounded off by a conclusion. Otherwise, they tend be left with a 'so what' type of feeling about your presentation. Don't just stop with your last research finding, but offer some kind of concluding statement, even if it's just a sentence or two.

▲ Use the conclusion to summarise facts

Many presentations will use the conclusion to summarise the facts and findings just presented, to highlight key points, and perhaps to synthesise knowledge from several different sources.

▲ Use the conclusion to make recommendations, if appropriate

In addition to summarising knowledge, the conclusion can be the place where you make recommendations based on that knowledge. For example, you might like to state what further studies are needed (especially if you are already doing them). Or you might like to make recommendations for changes in clinical practice, or other actions you think should be taken.

▲ Let the audience know when you're about to conclude the presentation

Warning your audience that the conclusion is coming gives them a chance to sit up and concentrate on what you have to say.

▲ Don't make your conclusion too long

If your conclusion goes on for too long, the audience will start to lose interest – in fact, if they were looking forward to a break they may become distinctly disgruntled. So limit the length of your conclusion to five to ten per cent of your talk. No one likes a long, drawn-out conclusion. Even worse is the 'bumpy landing', where the speaker keeps saying 'and finally', but the 'final' point is followed by another, and then another.

▲ Word your conclusion carefully and rehearse it well

Your last words should be memorable. Think about using some of the 'powerful' words mentioned in Chapter 9. To help you remember your conclusion, write it out word-for-word and practise it (but never read it from your notes on the actual day).

▲ Try some of these ideas for your conclusion

What you say will depend on the body of your talk, but here are a few ideas:

- Match your conclusion to your objectives for your talk.
- Refer back to your opening remarks (e.g. what was the aim of your study).
- Use a memorable quotation.
- Tell an anecdote or joke (but be careful here).
- Make a recommendation.
- Look at the future.

▲ Avoid an apologetic conclusion

However badly you feel the presentation has gone, never end in an apologetic manner. The audience may not have been riveted to the spot, but they will certainly take a worse view of what they've just heard if you end by saying, 'Well, I'm sorry I didn't have time to tell you more about …' or 'I hope you didn't find that too boring after this morning's exciting presentations'. The chances are they will not have noticed any minor slip-ups or omissions, so there's no point in your drawing attention to them.

8

Scripting your presentation

Your immediate response to the title of this section might well be 'Everyone knows you should never read a presentation, so surely you shouldn't write a script!' We understand your concerns, and agree that there are only a few circumstances in which you should actually read your presentation from a script (see below). However, that does not necessarily mean that you should not write it out in full. In fact, many speakers (both experienced and inexperienced) find it helpful to write out precisely what they plan to say, though they may not use those actual words when they give the talk.

▲ Decide whether you need a script for this particular presentation

It's definitely not compulsory to write a script. Some powerful presenters never write one. Others only do so for certain types of talk. A few would never dream of speaking without one. It's up to you.

▲ Writing it doesn't necessarily mean you will read from it

A few confident speakers use no notes at all. Many more give a polished talk, aided only by a few notes or even a one-page mind map. But when you see someone apparently speaking 'off the cuff', that doesn't necessarily mean their presentation hasn't been worked out in considerable detail in advance. Writing a script can be helpful, even if you don't refer to it on the day. In a few circumstances, it can be essential (see below).

▲ A script can give you confidence

Presidents and Prime Ministers use speechwriters to help them give a polished but apparently 'spontaneous' presentation (often aided by an unseen autocue). So why should we not emulate them by 'scripting' our presentations in advance? On the day, if you present it correctly, no one will know or care whether you have 'scripted' your presentation or not.

▲ A script can help you identify and overcome potential problems

Writing out your presentation in full allows you to:

- make sure that the length is just right
- reassure yourself that nothing has been missed out
- iron out problems of word choice
- show your presentation to a number of different colleagues without having to invite all of them to a rehearsal.

▲ A script can be useful in an emergency

A script also allows you to:

- have a backup to which you can refer if you 'freeze' with stage-fright on the day
- ask someone else to take your place in an emergency (e.g. if you are ill, or your flight is delayed).

▲ A script can also have other uses

Under specific circumstances, a script can fill additional functions. It enables you to:

- show your presentation to a translator if the meeting has simultaneous translation
- prepare a proceedings manuscript quickly and easily – you will already be halfway there.

▲ Normally, you never read from your script …

Just because you have written your presentation, it does not mean that you should read from it verbatim. Reading your presentation is likely to make it seem lifeless, and may undermine your authority and credibility as a presenter. However, as shown in the next tip, there are a few circumstances in which it *is* advisable to read your presentation from a script.

▲ ... Except in these three circumstances

It is advisable to read your presentation under the following circumstances:

- **If you are speaking in a language in which you are not confident.** Reading from a script will minimise errors and make your presentation more intelligible.
- **If the topic is legally or politically sensitive.** If what you say could have legal or political repercussions, it is wise to read from a script, which you can have checked by the relevant authorities beforehand.
- **If you are speaking on behalf of someone else.** You may occasionally be called upon to present someone else's data, in which case you will be a great deal more confident if you have a script.

▲ You don't have to memorise your talk word-for-word ...

Just because you have scripted your talk, it doesn't mean you will necessarily use the same words when you come to give it. A talk that is memorised parrot-fashion is likely to sound very flat. The important thing is to include everything you need to say in the script, to give you confidence. Then you can paraphrase as much as you like when you deliver it.

▲ ... But you might like to memorise a few telling phrases

Despite the advice against learning your talk word-for-word, there is no doubt that memorising key sections can be confidence-building. If you are not a naturally eloquent speaker, it may help you to memorise the key phrases from your introduction and conclusions, so that you can be confident of making coherent, powerful statements at the times when everyone will be listening hardest. There's more about introductions and conclusions in Chapters 5 and 7.

▲ Write for the ear, not the eye

When scripting your talk, remember that your words will eventually be spoken. Writing for the ear has to be simpler than writing for the eye. Rhythm is also more important. The tips in Chapter 9 will help you to write a talk that can be easily remembered and spoken.

9

Choosing and using words

Your choice of words and the way you combine them can make or break a presentation. In scientific presentations, we are aiming for technical accuracy, but we are also aiming to create a positive, powerful impression on the audience. The right choice of words can help us to achieve both aims.

▲ Stick to one idea per sentence

The golden rule is that a sentence should express a single thought. Often, if you write a long sentence, you will find that it contains more than one idea, and can be easily split into two sentences (see below). If you have a very small thought, don't be afraid to say a short sentence.

▲ Test your sentences for length

In scientific papers, sentences of 30 words or more are common. Yet, if you try to read these long sentences aloud, you will swiftly find yourself running out of breath or stumbling over complex constructions. Long sentences may be manageable in writing (if your audience is playing close attention), but in talks they are difficult for both the speaker and the listener. So, get into the habit of speaking in short sentences you can say in one breath.

▲ Vary sentence length

A presentation consisting only of eight-word sentences would sound like machine gun fire. A presentation consisting only of 30-word sentences would put the audience to sleep. Varying sentence length is more pleasant for the listener and helps to keep them alert and awake. Varying the pace of delivery and the type of material you're covering also helps to stop the audience falling asleep.

▲ Put powerful ideas in short, sharp sentences

Your key points should be presented in short, memorable sentences. In fact, some of the world's most memorable ideas have been expressed in very short sentences – 'Less is more', 'I have a dream', 'Ich bin ein Berliner'.

▲ Use active sentence constructions

Scientific writing tends to make use of passive constructions. Often this is in an attempt to avoid using personal pronouns and thereby to sound more impersonal. Thus, we may write 'the dose was titrated' instead of 'we titrated the dose'. Note that the passive voice is always longer. It usually sounds more boring. So why not stick with 'we titrated the dose', which is entirely acceptable in a formal presentation.

▲ Don't smother your verbs

A verb is smothered when it is turned into a noun and an extra verb added. Thus, 'we studied so-and-so' becomes 'a study was performed of so-and so'. 'We analysed' becomes 'an analysis was made' and so on. This kind of construction sounds pompous and will make you a wordy speaker. Try to get out of the habit.

▲ Use words and phrases you would use in everyday speech

Think carefully before you use any words that you would not use when having a conversation with somebody. For example, how often do you say 'advantageous' in everyday speech? There is no special vocabulary for presentations. You may use technical terms, but there's no harm in using everyday words for everyday things. Your vocabulary should be the same as if you are having a conversation with the audience, but avoid slang expressions (see next tip).

▲ Avoid slang and colloquialisms

It's quite likely your audience will include people who speak English as a second or third language. For this reason it's important to avoid slang expressions or colloquialisms they may not know. Say that something is 'never going to be successful', rather than 'we're on a hiding to nothing'. Say 'However fit you are, you can still suffer from altitude sickness' rather than 'You can be as fit as a butcher's dog and still suffer from altitude sickness'. Avoiding slang also helps to lend an air of professionalism to your presentation.

▲ Avoid unfamiliar jargon

Jargon may be described as 'the language of exclusion'. There's nothing wrong with technical terms – provided everyone in your audience understands them. The minute you use a word your audience doesn't know, you confuse them – they may feel patronised or insulted. So choose your technical terms carefully. If you're talking to doctors, say 'hypertension', but if you're talking to health service administrators, say 'high blood pressure'.

▲ Avoid unfamiliar abbreviations and acronyms

As with technical terms, think beforehand about which abbreviations and acronyms will be familiar to your audience. In general, stick to standard abbreviations that are well known to your audience (e.g. DNA or PCR for geneticists). If you repeat a long, tongue-tripping name frequently (e.g. cardiac insufficiency bisoprolol study), it's acceptable to explain the abbreviation (CIBIS) and then use it throughout your talk, but try not to do this for too many terms within a talk.

▲ Use your audience's language

One of the ways you can create empathy with your audience is to use their language. Sometimes the adjustments you may need to make are obvious – for example, if you're a scientist talking to the lay public, you need to use as few technical terms as possible. Sometimes the adjustments are more subtle. If you're talking to a technical audience outside your own speciality, it is useful to get a friendly expert to review your talk. They can help make sure you're using exactly the 'right' terminology, and the most up-to-date terms.

▲ Add a few 'buzzwords'

Provided you know what you're doing, you can add to your rapport with the audience by using a few words or phrases that you know will attract attention and establish you as an 'insider'. For example, if you're talking to health economists about clinical matters, bringing in terms like 'evidence-based healthcare' and 'cost-effectiveness' will help to attract their attention.

▲ But avoid 'turn-off' language

You need to know what kind of language keeps your audience happy, but you also need to beware of language that 'turns them off'. For example, if you're a business person talking to technical people, beware of using business slang or vogue phrases such as 'ball-park figure'.

▲ Use words precisely

In technical presentations, it's vital to use terms precisely. Sloppy use of language could confuse your audience. Use the most precise word for what you're trying to describe. For example, why 'quantify' or 'evaluate' something when you can 'measure', 'count', 'estimate' or 'calculate' it? Of course, you could use the broader word to cover more than one step.

▲ Beware of unfamiliar words

One of the benefits of sticking to simple, everyday language for simple, everyday things is that you do not inadvertently misuse words, and thereby undermine your credibility. If you're not sure what a word means, don't use it.

▲ Choose your 'proving' words carefully according to strength

Prove is the strongest word we can use about scientific findings (though it can rarely be used in biomedical studies, which mainly focus on probability rather than certainty). Here are some others, in descending order of strength. Think about which one matches the strength of your conclusions. Can you think of any others?

- show
- demonstrate
- indicate
- suggest
- imply

▲ Be cautious …

Very little is incontrovertible in science. It is accepted and appropriate to use 'hedging' words such as:

- may be
- might be
- could be
- probably
- possibly

and so on.

▲ … But not excessively so

However, do not 'hedge' so much that you show little confidence in your results.

- *These results suggest that the cause of X is Y* is acceptable.
- *These results suggest that the cause of X may be Y* is weaker, but (may possibly be) appropriate if you are being very cautious.
- *These results suggest the possibility that the cause of X may ultimately be found to be Y* is ridiculously over-cautious, not to mention pompous.

▲ Be positive – unless you want to deliberately create doubt

Research shows that people find positive statements easier to understand than negative ones. Thus, 'in most patients, pain was relieved by day six' is easier to understand than 'most patients did not experience pain beyond day six'. However, the positive or negative statement of the same finding can have a different influence on people's perceptions. Compare 'the procedure has a 90 per cent success rate' with 'the procedure has a 10 per cent failure rate'. Which statement would encourage you to undergo the procedure? Thus, you can use negative statements as part of the process of countering or undermining an argument.

▲ Use 'you' or 'we' language where appropriate

You will notice that a lot of this book is written in 'you' language because we are talking to you, the reader. We may not know your names as individuals, but we know that it's you we are trying to reach. The same thing can apply to presentations: 'The techniques described in this presentation will help you to manage diabetes more effectively and more economically.' Using 'we' can also help to create empathy: 'We need to find ways of treating more patients, more quickly.' However, beware of making the presentation too personal, otherwise the audience will feel under pressure. Varying 'you' with 'health professional' or 'doctor' will take some of the pressure off. Never use 'you' when you are about to explain the error of the audience's ways. 'Studies show that we are only prescribing ACE inhibitors to 50 per cent of eligible patients with heart failure' is less aggressive than 'studies show that you are only prescribing ...'. 'Studies show that 50 per cent of eligible heart failure patients are not receiving ACE inhibitors' is more neutral still.

▲ Use 'powerful' words

When you reach an important part of your presentation, highlight its importance with 'powerful' words such as:

- interesting
- fascinating
- unusual
- decisive
- exciting
- new
- critical
- urgent
- compelling
- vital
- crucial
- key
- pivotal
- convincing.

Think about using these and other powerful words more often in your presentations. We are often so concerned with seeming professional that we avoid using the obvious potent words and go instead for their watered-down equivalents. You're not writing advertising copy, but that doesn't mean you can't effectively borrow some of the language that is used to sell cars and soap powder. Even sophisticated listeners are susceptible to the power of emotive words.

▲ Avoid foreign or Latin words and phrases

A presentation is rarely the place to show off your knowledge of foreign words or phrases or classical Latin or Greek. It's confusing for the audience and implies that if they don't know those words or phrases, they must be less clever than you. So, prefer 'never despair' to 'nil desperandum', and talk about a 'choice of treatments' instead of an 'armamentarium'. You can, of course, use the Latin names of organisms.

▲ Be careful with clichés

The usual advice about clichés is to avoid them ('like the plague'). Generally I would agree with this. Clichés ('the gold standard treatment for …') often sound boring and pompous. However, there may also be occasions on which you would like to use just one or two, to establish a bond of common language with your audience.

10

Learn from professional orators

You may not think that you have much to learn from politicians, especially those for whom you would not dream of voting. Yet, next time a political speech is reported on TV, listen carefully. You may well hear some of the following rhetorical devices, first used by orators in ancient Greece to make their speeches more powerful and interesting. Nowadays they're most often used by politicians, lawyers and experienced presenters. Judiciously incorporating such devices into your own presentations will help you to establish your reputation as a polished and professional speaker.

▲ Alliteration

Alliteration describes a phrase in which two or more words begin with the same sound, such as 'diabetes can be a distressing and debilitating condition'. Alliterative phrases tend to add emphasis and to stick in the audience's mind. They can be used anywhere in your talk, and combined with many of the other devices listed below.

▲ Metaphor

A metaphor is an implied comparison that transfers the properties of one thing to another. Unlike a simile (see below), you don't say something is *like* something else, but speak as if it *is* something else. 'An iron curtain has descended across the continent' (Winston Churchill). 'Heart failure is a maze.' 'Stroke prevention is real tiger country.'

▲ Simile

Simile is used when you say something is *like* something else. 'Trying to manage people is like herding cats.' 'A computer is like a filing cabinet.'

▲ Rhetorical question

A rhetorical question is used for effect – the audience isn't expected to answer. Rhetorical questions alert the audience to the importance of the question – but you shouldn't make them wait too long before you provide them with the answer, or they'll lose interest. Rhetorical questions often work well as introductions or transitions, or occasionally as conclusions. 'How do cells know when to start dividing? And how do they know when to stop? In this presentation we'll look at …'

▲ Antithesis

Anthithesis describes the opposition or contrast of ideas in a balanced or parallel construction. 'They died that we might live.' 'It was the best of times, it was the worst of times, it was the age of foolishness …' (Charles Dickens). It's easy to create your own antithesis – just pick two opposites (words or phrases), and write a sentence with one of the opposites in each half. 'We're so good at diagnosing this disease, and so bad at treating it.'

▲ Hyperbole

Hyperbole refers to exaggeration for effect. 'His presentation lasted for aeons.' 'If you call, I'll be there at the speed of light.' 'A horse, a horse, my kingdom for a horse.' It can be used occasionally in technical presentations, as long as you're sure you're not going to confuse anyone.

▲ Litotes

Litotes describes an ironical understatement, in which you deny the opposite of the thing you would like to emphasise. Confused? You won't be when you see some examples. 'This is no small problem' (meaning 'this is a big problem'). 'It is not inconceivable that …' (meaning 'it is conceivable that'). Use this device sparingly, for fear of confusing your listeners, especially those whose first language is not English.

▲ Paradox

A paradoxical statement is one that at first sight seems opposed to common sense, but which is in fact true. 'The more people diet, the fatter they get.' 'Youth is wasted on the young.'

▲ Oxymoron

An oxymoron is a special kind of paradox in which two apparently contradictory words or phrases are juxtaposed. 'Make haste slowly.' 'Be cruel to be kind.'

▲ Tautology

Tautology is the repetition of an idea in a different word, phrase or sentence. People sometimes say 'that's a tautology' when they mean to be critical of someone who has thoughtlessly used more than one word to say the same thing, as in 'at the present moment in time' or 'try and endeavour'. I would certainly discourage you from using it in writing. Yet, in speech, it is a legitimate technique to add emphasis. 'With malice towards none, with charity for all' (Abraham Lincoln).

▲ Repetition

You can repeat a key phrase at intervals throughout your presentation, to underline a key idea. A classic example would be Martin Luther King's 'I have a dream' speech. Another use of repetition is in parallel statements within one section or one sentence of your presentation. 'Tough on crime, tough on the causes of crime' (Tony Blair). 'We know how this disease develops. We know how to diagnose it. We know how to treat it. What we do not know is how to prevent it.' This last example is also an example of climax (see below).

▲ Climax

Climax describes a series of statements building up to a peak of intensity. 'I came, I saw, I conquered' (Julius Caesar) is an example of climax (and also of parallel structure and alliteration).

▲ Play on words

Some memorable phrases rely on the use of similar sounding words or double meanings. 'The lady's not for turning' (Margaret Thatcher, referring to *The Lady's not for Burning* by Christopher Fry).

▲ Use the rule of three

For some reason, people find things that come in threes particularly memorable. From time immemorial, public figures have used the 'rule of three' in their speeches. Julius Caesar again – 'I came, I saw, I conquered'. Winston Churchill – 'I have nothing to offer you but blood, sweat and tears'.

Did you notice anything odd about the last example? If you did, congratulations! What Churchill actually said was 'blood, sweat, tears and toil' – but only about one person in a hundred remembers the 'toil', because of the power of the rule of three.

The rule of three is also widely used in advertising – 'A Mars a day helps you work, rest and play'.

11

Slide preparation: basic principles

Most of the tips in this section apply whether you are using computer-generated slides, traditional 35 mm slides, or overhead projector acetates. Although we've made the assumption that you are probably using PowerPoint, the commonest presentation program, the same principles apply to other software.

▲ Don't assume that slides are compulsory

Although most biomedical presentations focus on data and therefore require numerous graphs and tables, remember that not every talk falls into this category. Some of the most effective presentations we have seen depended purely on the words, voice and physical presence of the speaker to communicate a powerful message. If you are talking about your own experiences, or making an impassioned plea for a cause, consider dispensing with the scientific slides and speaking simply from the heart instead.

▲ Think about the purpose of each slide

Slides can serve many functions. For example, they can:

- show data – the most obvious function, but not the only one
- provide reinforcement – for example, slides that outline a talk or state conclusions
- attract attention – for example, a striking or unexpected picture.

The most effective presentations are those that contain some of each kind of slide.

▲ Each slide should have a single overall message

In your own mind, it should be possible to sum up the point of each slide in a single sentence. For example, 'this graph shows response rates at one week' or 'these are the three main conclusions from our research'. Each graph or table should tell a single coherent story, whether it is a graph, table, text slide or picture. Of course, it is possible for messages to be broken down into subpoints, but they should all centre on the same theme.

▲ Don't try to merge slides

Don't try to combine unlike types of information on the same slide just to cut down on the total number of slides. For example, it may at first seem like a good idea to display a graph with three bullet points alongside it summing up what's in the graph. But why have both picture and words? You could make those same three points in your talk, leaving the audience to focus on the graph itself.

▲ Limit the number of slides

We've all seen presentations that used so many slides the audience could barely register what was being shown before the speaker moved on to the next. No matter how much data you have, it is possible to be selective. You need to restrict the number of slides to avoid overloading the brains of your audience. With simple slides, you may be able to show as many as two per minute. The minute you begin to show more complex slides, limit yourself to no more than one a minute.

▲ The more complicated the slides, the fewer there should be

Usually, you will have a mixture of types of slides – as a rule of thumb, try to have no more than 30 slides for a 20-minute talk. If you use the 'build' feature of PowerPoint for text or graphic slides, it's the completed slide that counts towards the total. But don't do a build on every slide (see below).

▲ Use a consistent orientation

Slides should be in either landscape or portrait orientation – never a mixture of both, as this is disorientating for the audience.

▲ Landscape orientation is safest

Most projection screens are sized for landscape orientation, and this format is also the most adaptable for showing graphs and tables. Although PowerPoint and other slide programs can create slides with a portrait format, it's wisest to stick to the default, which is always landscape. We've seen presentations in which the top and bottom of portrait-format slides were cut off when projected on a 'landscape' screen.

▲ Give each slide its own informative title …

All graphs, diagrams, tables and text slides should have their own title. This reinforces the slide's key message, and helps the audience to follow the structure of the talk. It can also be very valuable to you if you lose the thread of what you're saying.

▲ … But avoid using titles on photos unless they're really necessary

Photos (e.g. radiographs, histology slides, or photos of people or places) usually look better if they occupy the whole screen, without a title.

▲ Only number PowerPoint slides if you are using them in parallel with handouts

PowerPoint will let you give each slide a number, but there's no point in doing this during a typical conference presentation – it's just a distraction for the audience. However, in a teaching situation, if the audience are following the talk on handouts, it may be appropriate to show the number on the slides so that they can find their place in the handouts.

▲ Use PowerPoint templates to enhance consistency

It's possible to build up a PowerPoint slide from a blank screen, adding colours, fonts, logos and other features 'from scratch'. However, PowerPoint also contains 'design templates' – predesigned formats and colour schemes that can be applied to any presentation to give it a co-ordinated look. You can use PowerPoint's existing templates, modify them, or design your own.

▲ Choose a template consistent with your subject matter

PowerPoint offers a wide range of slide templates. Some are suitable for scientific presentations, whereas others are more suited to business, or school or hobby presentations. Have a look at the full range to see if there is one that looks appropriate for your presentation.

▲ Avoid templates with fussy backgrounds

A background with complicated graphics may be appropriate for a presentation with mainly text slides. But in science, you're likely to have some complex graphs and tables to present, which would look confusing on a fussy background. So choose a template with a 'clean' background – typically monochrome, or with just a simple gradation of colour.

▲ If necessary, background graphics can be omitted from all slides …

If you find you like a particular template, but it has background graphics, PowerPoint allows you to omit them (Format, Background).

▲ … Or just selected slides

If you have mainly text slides and want to use a template with a background graphic, and just a couple of graphs, you could omit the background graphic from the graphs.

▲ Check to see if your institution has its own template

You may find that your university department, research institution or company has a standard template that you can use. This could save you time and trouble, and lends an air of authority to your presentation. However, remember that when you leave you will no longer be entitled to use an institutional template.

▲ You can design your own template

PowerPoint allows you to design your own template – useful if you cannot find something that suits your needs exactly. You can base your design on an existing template, or start from scratch using PowerPoint's basic tools. Don't forget to save it alongside the other templates. Don't go down this route if you are short of time, have no eye for design, or hate messing around with computers.

▲ You can have a template designed for you

You can get a template designed especially for you by a specialist slide designer – look on the Internet or in your local Yellow Pages for slide production companies.

▲ You can download additional PowerPoint templates from the Internet

If none of the templates that come with your PowerPoint program suit you, there are various Internet sources that you can try:

- Microsoft's own website offers occasional new templates.
- Commercial companies offer templates for sale.
- Free downloads are also available from companies or amateur enthusiasts.

▲ Don't forget that you can change the colours of templates

If you like a template but don't like the colour scheme, it's possible to alter it. Go to Format, then Slide colour scheme, then choose Custom. You may need some trial and error to come up with a combination of colours that works.

▲ Use a light background for a light room

If the room in which the slide will be projected is not going to be completely darkened – for example, a small seminar room – choose a light background colour for your slides. White, light blue or light tan work well. On a light background, the text should be dark, e.g. dark blue or black. Bullets can be in a contrasting colour, e.g. dark red.

▲ For darkened lecture halls, use a dark background colour

For a typical conference situation – a large, darkened room with no natural light – choose a dark background colour, e.g. navy blue. Text and bullets should be light, e.g. yellow or white.

▲ Avoid black backgrounds

For a dark background, don't choose black – it doesn't project well. Dark blue is a safe choice (see below). Dark green also works, but may have 'ecological' associations. Dark brown works as well, but its associations may not be right for science – though we once saw it used to great effect in a presentation about the chemistry of chocolate.

▲ Don't be afraid to follow a conventional 'scientific' colour scheme

If you're unsure what colour combination to use, don't be afraid to use the conventional 'scientific' format, which you've no doubt seen dozens of times in other people's presentations. It's widely used because it works. A standard combination (for a darkened room) is:

- dark blue background (could fade top-to-bottom or diagonally)
- white text
- yellow bullets
- yellow title.

▲ Prefer a sans serif font

Sans serif fonts (those without little 'tails' on the letters) are easier to read when projected on a distant screen. Examples of suitable sans serif fonts include Arial, Helvetica and Tahoma. Serif typefaces like Times New Roman are best avoided in slides (though they work well when used at a small font size as in printed books and newspapers). Check whether you are happy with the default font used with your chosen PowerPoint template. If you don't think it looks right, you can change it. This is much more efficient than changing the font on each slide one at a time.

▲ Allow plenty of time for proofreading your slides

It's mortifying to notice a mistake on your slides for the first time when you're in the middle of your talk. It's even worse if the mistake is important (e.g. a decimal point in the wrong place). So allow plenty of time to proofread your slides.

▲ Remember you are not selling technology

Some people really enjoy the process of preparing their slides, and want to use every technological trick in the book. Others see PowerPoint and other programs simply as a means to an end. If you are a technophile, by all means enjoy yourself, but don't overload the audience with gimmicks just for the sake of it – remember that you are talking about science, not selling presentation software.

▲ Keep your audience's expectations in mind

If you want to 'fit in' with your peer group, it's important to meet their expectations of what a presentation should be like. Scientific audiences, for example, are not easily impressed by technological wizardry. So, only use devices such as animations, fancy transitions, or other PowerPoint 'bells and whistles' if they are genuinely appropriate to the subject matter and actually add something to the presentation. Otherwise you run the risk of being dismissed as a 'lightweight'.

▲ Don't overdo the slide effects

It's possible to give a perfectly professional slide presentation without using any of the special effects that PowerPoint offers. There's no denying that some effects such as builds, transitions and animations can add interest and help to draw attention to the key points of your talk. Think carefully about the overall impression, however. The more effects you use, the more your talk will look like a PowerPoint demonstration rather than a scientific presentation.

▲ You can use builds to underline the structure of your talk ...

Builds are a good way to demonstrate the development of an argument, or describe steps in a process. For example, you could use a build in your conclusions, so that the audience can focus on one point at a time. Or you could add lines to a graph, one by one.

▲ ... But don't use a build on every slide

If you use them for every slide, they lose their impact, and audiences will quickly become bored with the device. Reserve builds for when they're really relevant and useful in focusing the audience's attention on one key point at a time.

▲ Remember that equipment may limit the use of some effects

Bear in mind that what works well on your home or office computer may not work as perfectly on borrowed equipment. For example, older, slower computers may not be able to display video well.

▲ Poor photos make poor slides

Remember that images projected on a large screen lose some of their definition. So, if something is quite difficult to see on your computer screen, it will probably disappear altogether when projected.

▲ Transition effects are strictly optional

It's perfectly permissible to switch from one slide to another with no transition effects at all. If you don't like transitions, don't feel under pressure to use them just because other people do.

▲ If you do use transitions, don't use any more than three types within a presentation

If you try to add variety to your talk by using the whole range of transitions that PowerPoint offers, the audience are likely to find it distracting or annoying. So, we suggest that you limit yourself to a maximum of three different effects.

▲ Don't use the random transitions feature in a scientific presentation

The random transitions feature may be fun, but is inappropriate in a scientific presentation. As always, you want the audience to focus on the content of your talk, not to be distracted by wondering 'Which transition will it be next?'

▲ Match transition effects to key transitions in the talk

One way of using transitions effectively is to match them to the psychological effect you want to create. For example:

- wipes are a safe, straightforward way of switching from one slide to another
- dissolves can be used to indicate time passing
- fade to black can be used to separate major sections of your talk.

12

Slide preparation: titles

One of the hallmarks of professionally produced slides is the effective use of titles. Slide titles help your audience (and you!) to follow the structure of the talk. Applying a consistent title style to all your slides helps them to look clean, clear and uncluttered.

▲ Limit titles to two lines maximum – just one if possible

Every slide (except photos) should have its own title. Although PowerPoint allows titles of more than two lines (it simply reduces the size of the font to make it fit), this is rarely necessary. The ideal title is just one line – two is permissible, but don't make all your titles two-liners.

▲ Titles can be made to fit by deleting waste words

Titles can be made to fit into one or two lines by deleting waste words. Thus 'A comparison of grottomycin with scabicillin in acute sinusitis' would become 'Grottomycin vs. scabicillin in acute sinusitis' or 'Acute sinusitis: grottomycin vs. scabicillin' (which would save you a couple of characters if space is tight).

▲ Titles need not be complete sentences

Remember that titles don't have to be complete sentences – that usually gives the audience too much to read. Phrases are better – edit out words like 'a study on' or 'a comparison of' – to a scientific audience it will be obvious that it is a study or a comparison.

▲ If you need space for just one or two more characters, stretch the title placeholder

When you have edited out every waste word you possibly can, you can make space for just one or two characters by adjusting the size of the standard PowerPoint title placeholder. This will allow you to make titles fit neatly onto just one or two lines, but don't abuse this technique (i.e. don't take the text right up to the edge of the slide).

▲ Avoid 'continued' titles

If, even after rigorous editing, you have too much text for one slide, you'll need to split it into two or more slides. You might then be tempted to head the slide something like *Conclusions (cont'd)* or *Conclusions I, II and III.* This is not particularly helpful to the audience, and looks unprofessional. It's usually possible to break down the content into logical units and title them accordingly. Thus, you might have *'Conclusions – primary outcomes', 'Conclusions – secondary outcomes'* and *'Conclusions – safety and tolerability'.*

▲ Don't use full stops at the end of slide titles

A professional slide designer will never use a full stop at the end of a title, even if it is a complete sentence. They look fine without – it's the modern style of punctuation.

▲ Avoid putting titles in all capitals

You might be tempted to put your slide title in capitals to make it stand out. There are two good reasons to avoid this, however:

- Text is harder to read when it's all in capitals.
- Capitals take up more space than lower case letters – space that you will probably need when trying to make the title fit onto one or two lines.

▲ Use 'sentence case' for titles

The most convenient, modern style for titles is 'sentence case' – that is, the first letter of the title is capitalised as are the first letters of proper names, cities and countries, titles of institutions (e.g. University of Oxford), generic names of organisms, etc. – as in a normal sentence.

▲ Avoid 'title case'

The alternative to 'sentence case' is 'title case', in which you also capitalise the first letters of all the important words, but don't capitalise 'small' words like 'a', 'the' and 'with'. Avoid this, unless you want to give yourself unnecessary work to do – although PowerPoint allows you to highlight text and change it to 'title case', you will have to remember to do it, and inconsistencies are bound to arise.

13

Slide preparation: text

You will probably have some slides that are text only. Rigorous editing and attention to detail will help you to make your text slides more readable, polished and professional.

▲ Don't use text slides if there is an alternative way of presenting the data

If you can use a graph, table, diagram or photograph instead of text, do so – too much text is boring for the audience. All too often, text slides just echo the speaker's words instead of adding something new to the talk.

▲ Limit text slides to no more than seven lines

Keeping text slides to no more than seven lines of text (plus the title) is a good rule of thumb for readability. It's often said that the average person can hold seven items at once in their short-term memory. But even seven lines is quite a lot to take in at once – there's no harm in having slides that are shorter than seven lines!

▲ Use bullet points rather than continuous text

Unless you are quoting a full sentence from somewhere else (e.g. a definition, or a quote from a famous scientist), try to avoid putting whole paragraphs of text on the screen. Breaking text down into bullet points allows you to break ideas into logical chunks. It also frees you from the need to write full sentences, which means you can be more concise.

▲ Limit bullet points to one line wherever possible

Most bullet points should be no longer than one line (which, if you follow the seven lines principle, means no more than seven bullet points to a slide). You can help to work towards this ideal by editing out all waste words and using abbreviated phrases rather than full sentences (see below).

▲ There's no need to make bullet points into full sentences

Just because you speak in full sentences, there's no reason why your slides should represent exactly what you say. After all, you won't be reading from your slides (or at least we hope you won't). The words are merely there as reinforcement for the audience (and to jog your memory if you get stuck). Words and phrases are easier for the audience to take in, and take up a lot less space than full sentences.

▲ Use sentence case in text slides

Text slides usually look best if they are written in sentence case, i.e. each bullet point (whether a word, phrase or sentence) starts with a capital letter, but continues in lower case (except for proper nouns, names, etc. which are capitalised in the normal way).

▲ Don't mix full sentences and phrases in the same bullet-point list

If you do use full sentences, make sure every item in the list is a full sentence – don't mix sentences up with words and phrases.

▲ Edit the text of bullet points to make the structure of each item consistent

You can help to create a pleasing, professional effect by editing the text of your bullet points, so that similar items follow a similar structure. It's easiest to understand what we mean by looking at an example. Let's say we have a slide entitled 'Effects of stress at work'. Your first idea for the slide might be something like:

- Tiredness causes loss of concentration when performing difficult tasks.
- Poor motivation results from depression and anxiety.
- Stress-related illnesses can result in poor attendance because of sick leave.
- Alienation of colleagues can arise due to irritability and anger.

You'll notice a couple of things about this bullet-point list. It is written in full sentences (which is unnecessary), and the structure of the individual items is inconsistent (sometimes we have effect–cause, sometimes cause–effect). How about changing it into something like:

- Tiredness – loss of concentration
- Depression – lack of motivation
- Illness – poor attendance
- Irritability – impaired relationships.

Your spoken words would fill in any gaps.

▲ Consider using text tables to highlight relationships

Don't forget that tables don't always have to contain figures – you can fill them with key words instead to show the relationships between ideas. For example, the text above could become:

Effects of stress at work

Symptom	Effect on performance
Tiredness	Loss of concentration
Depression	Lack of motivation
Illness	Poor attendance
Irritability	Impaired relationships

▲ Simple graphic devices can also be used to display text

In addition to text tables, simple graphics can also be used to display text in an interesting way. Again, the objective is to highlight the relationships between ideas. You can use the drawing tools, or save time by using simple clipart, adapted to suit your purposes. An example is shown below – there must be dozens of other ways in which you could display the same material.

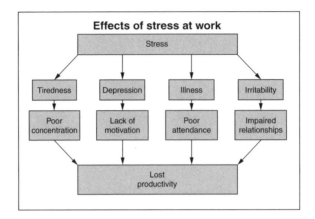

▲ Highlight key points on text slides with colour, rather than bold

Colour usually works better than bold for highlighting key points on text slides, as the bold effect may be lost on projection.

▲ In text slides, reserve italics for the Latin names of organisms and Latin phrases

Italics aren't a good way of adding emphasis – they actually tend to make what is italicised fade into the background rather than stand out. So keep italics for their technical use, i.e. for organisms, e.g. *Saccharomyces carlsbergiensis*, and in necessary Latin phrases such as *in vitro* and *in vivo*.

▲ Try not to have all text slides

With many scientific presentations, there will be plenty of graphs, tables and charts to show. With others, it may seem as if your entire presentation is dominated by text slides. Obviously, you have to do your best with the material at hand, but try to think of ways in which you can make the text more interesting. For example, links between ideas could be expressed as a simple diagram, or a series of linked shapes containing key words (see above).

14

Slide preparation: tables

Tables are a common feature of scientific presentations. These tips will help you produce tables that are easy for the audience to understand. The ideal is to design the table so that the audience can go straight to the critical data.

▲ Give each table a slide to itself

Don't attempt to fit more than one table on a slide. Even if the table is very simple, it deserves a slide to itself.

▲ Do not use tables if the data could be better shown in a graph

Generally speaking, graphs get their message across to an audience more effectively than tables. So, if the data could be given as either a graph or a table, pick the graph.

▲ Use tables to display relationships between discontinuous variables

Some types of data don't lend themselves to being graphed. For example, if you want to show baseline data for two groups of participants in a clinical trial, such as sex, age, weight, smoking history and concomitant diseases, you will need a table.

▲ Use tables when the audience need to see exact values

Sometimes, the audience will be more interested in the exact values for certain parameters than in comparing them between groups. In such a case, a table might be more appropriate than a graph. However, remember that it is sometimes possible to add key numbers to line graphs and bar charts, if you think it will help the audience.

▲ Keep tables in talks simpler than those used in scientific papers

In a paper, the audience has time to look carefully at a table and to come back to it more than once if they need to. With a slide, the table is on the screen for a short time – usually less than a minute – and then gone forever. Tables in scientific presentations should therefore be less complex than those you might use in a paper.

▲ Remember you can use ultra-simple tables that would be unacceptable in a paper

In scientific papers, editors try to keep the number of tables and graphs within certain limits, in order to restrict the overall length of papers. Editors will usually ask you to edit out a table with, say, two columns and three rows. In presentations, there is no such restriction. So, if you think it would help the audience, use a table.

▲ Follow the five by seven rule

A good rule of thumb (for landscape slides) is to make your tables not more than five columns across, not more than seven rows down.

▲ Organise the table so the comparisons are made from left to right

It's more natural for readers to make comparisons crosswise rather than downwards, and (in Western cultures at least) the natural thing to do is to read from left to right.

▲ Do not give audiences too many numbers to take in at once

Choose units that eliminate unnecessary zeros and consider rounding numbers up or down to make them simpler to understand.

▲ Remember that you can highlight key points in tables

You can highlight important rows or columns by putting the numbers in bold, or in a different colour, or applying a background tint to the whole row or column. With electronic slides, you can highlight different parts of the table in turn as you talk the audience through them.

▲ Keep column headings short

Try to stop column headings running on to a second line. If necessary, use abbreviations and define them at the bottom of the table, or tell the audience what they mean.

▲ Make sure you include units of measure, where appropriate

Column and row headings should include units of measure (usually the International System of Units – SI), usually in brackets to the right of the variable being measured, e.g. Weight (kg). SI abbreviations don't need to be defined (see below).

▲ Define non-SI abbreviations, if necessary

SI abbreviations can always be used without definition. In contrast to papers, where you usually have to spell out any non-SI abbreviations the first time they are used, in presentations you can use your common sense about what the audience will recognise. So there's no need to spell out abbreviations that you are sure will be instantly familiar to your audience – for example, PCR (polymerase chain reaction) for geneticists, CABG (coronary artery bypass graft) for cardiologists.

▲ Be consistent about capitalisation of row and column headings

If you look at professionally produced slides, you will see that they are consistent in their use of capitals between and within slides. A good, easy-to-follow rule is to capitalise the first letter of all column and row headings. All proper names and genus names should also start with a capital letter, of course.

▲ Avoid footnotes in tables as far as possible

Footnotes are commonplace in tables prepared for papers. However, in a presentation, the audience doesn't really have time to try to take in the footnotes as well as the table. Some footnotes may occasionally be necessary, e.g. spelling out an unfamiliar abbreviation or giving the reference to the paper in which someone else's data originally appeared, but try to keep them to the minimum possible.

▲ Give row headings and subheadings a logical order

Rather than just put your row headings down in the order you first thought of, think about which order will make the data easiest to interpret.

▲ Indent subheadings where necessary

Indenting row subheadings will make the structure of the table easier to understand. For example:

Drug costs
   Anti-emetics
   Sedatives
Administration costs
   Disposables
   Physician time
   Nursing time

▲ Use only meaningful decimal places

Ask yourself how accurately you measured each variable. For means, do not give more than one decimal place above that in the original measurements. Consider rounding values for simplicity.

▲ Be consistent with decimal places

Use the same number of decimal places in all values for one variable. Use the same number of decimal places in standard deviations, standard errors or confidence intervals as in the mean.

▲ Use percentages where appropriate, but consider giving the raw data too

The use of percentages is particularly helpful when sample size varies between groups.

▲ You can give the raw data and percentages in the same column

For the reader's convenience, if the sample size varies, it is often appropriate to include both numbers and percentages in the same column. The percentages can come in brackets after the raw data.

▲ Do not leave cells blank

Leaving cells blank leaves the reader guessing – was the value zero, or was it just not successfully measured? A typical style is:

0.0 the value was zero
–   the value was not measured or is not given for some other reason.

▲ You can indicate statistical significance with *P* values or footnote indicators

You may want to give *P* values in a separate column. Alternatively, you can save space if you use asterisks, defined in footnotes. A standard series is *P<0.05; **P<0.01; ***P<0.001.

▲ Check and re-check your numbers

Make sure columns that are supposed to add up to 100% do so. Make sure that all parts of the sample are accounted for. It is distracting for the audience if they spot a discrepancy.

▲ Apply this editing checklist to your tables:

• Could/should you have used a graph instead?
• Are there no more than five columns and seven rows (if landscape)?
• Is the layout clear and uncomplicated?
• Does it have an appropriate title?
• Are key data highlighted?
• Are there any excessive decimal places?
• Are there any unnecessary footnotes?
• Are abbreviations obvious or explained?
• Are sources of data credited?
• Is irrelevant detail avoided?
• Are standard deviation (SD), confidence interval (CI) and *P* values included where appropriate?
• Do columns add up correctly?

15

Slide preparation: general hints for graphs and charts

Graphs and charts are one of the most effective ways to show relationships between data or ideas – but it's easy to get carried away and overload them with information. We've all seen presentations in which complex graphs or incomprehensible charts have flowed one after another in a continuous stream. Here's how to make sure your audience is enlightened rather than exhausted by graphical information.

▲ If in doubt, prefer graphs and charts to tables

When either a graph or a table would be appropriate, choose the graph. Graphs are quicker to understand at a glance than tables, so if the same data could be presented equally well with a graph or a table, choose the graph.

▲ Redraw graphs and charts in papers, rather than scanning them

If you are short of time, it's tempting to scan graphs from published papers and use them in presentations. This strategy should be used only as a last resort, for several reasons:

- It leads to inconsistency, which looks unprofessional.
- You will end up with black writing on a white background, which will probably be inconsistent with the rest of your slides.
- Text and symbols will often be too small.

- Strictly speaking, you need copyright permission from the original journal and the author to reproduce graphs exactly, whereas if you redraw them you can simply acknowledge the source of the original data.

▲ If possible, draw graphs and charts using PowerPoint's tools

PowerPoint allows you to draw graphs and charts with a minimum of trouble using raw data entered into a datasheet. You can also import Excel spreadsheets and convert them into PowerPoint graphs. Using the PowerPoint tools is the simplest way to make a professional-looking graph – provided, of course, that you have access to the original data or can easily obtain it by measuring a graph from someone else's paper.

▲ If you don't have the original data, graphs can be redrawn from a scanned image

If you do not have the original dataset, or it's too difficult to work out co-ordinates from a published graph, there is an alternative approach. You can scan in the graph, position it on the slide, and then draw over the parts you want using the drawing features in PowerPoint. You then delete the original scanned image, leaving you with the same graph, but with the colours and background of your choice.

▲ Use PowerPoint's graphing features in preference to its drawing tools

The disadvantages of using Powerpoint's drawing tools to produce a graph, in comparison with its graphing tools, are:

- drawing is time-consuming and fiddly
- you will have many decisions to make about line thickness, symbols, etc., which PowerPoint would otherwise make automatically
- you will have to learn a lot about PowerPoint's drawing features in order to obtain a professional result
- small changes made to a 'drawn' graph can have major knock-on effects, whereas when you change something in a PowerPoint graph, the program automatically makes the necessary adjustments to the rest of the graph with the minimum of fuss.

▲ Add error bars using the graphing tools, rather than drawing them

Note that if you add drawn items (e.g. error bars) to a graph prepared using the graphing tools, any changes to the graph will result in your having to move the drawn object. When you use the graphing tools, if you change the datasheet, the error bars are adjusted to reflect your changes.

16

Slide preparation: line graphs and scatter plots

These tips will help you to give line graphs and scatter plots a consistent, professional look.

▲ Put the continuous variable on the *x* axis

In line graphs, the convention is to put an independent and continuous variable – for example, time or concentration – on the *x* axis, and the dependent variable – for example, a measure of treatment effect – on the *y* axis.

▲ Limit the number of lines

If, as usually happens, a graph is on the screen for a minute or less, it is hard for audiences to take in the meaning at each line, so restrict the number of lines, even more than you would in graphs appearing in a printed paper or a poster. The rule should be not more than three to five lines (depending on whether the lines cross).

▲ Make sure that graph lines are thicker than the axes

The lines of the graph are where you want the audience to focus their attention, so check that they are thicker than the axes.

▲ Take care to use strong colours

Colour combinations that look attractive on your computer screen may look washed out and faded when projected, and it may become difficult to distinguish between colours. If in doubt, go for colours that seem a little bright – they will be 'toned down' on screen. Ideally, test your colour choices by projecting your slides under lighting conditions similar to those that will be used on the day.

▲ Avoid using red and green lines together on the same line graph

You might think that red and green would make a nice, easily distinguished colour contrast. Unfortunately, however, five per cent of men are red–green colour blind, so avoid putting red and green lines together on the same graph.

▲ Avoid broken lines – use solid colour instead

In papers, broken (dotted or dashed) lines are often used in graphs because the paper is printed in black and white. In slides, however, you always have colour, which is much easier for audiences to interpret. So, avoid broken lines on graphs, and if you are converting a graph that previously appeared in a paper to a slide, replace broken lines with solid, coloured ones.

▲ Don't use keys if lines can easily be labelled

If colour keys are used, the audience has to look in two different places to obtain the important message of the slide. When you can do so without making the slide impossibly messy, label the lines themselves instead of using a key.

▲ Add statistical information to line graphs where appropriate

Don't forget that you can add P values at appropriate points to show differences between groups at specified time points.

▲ Ensure that the graph lines fill most of the slide

Check that your axes are not too long compared with the graph content – in order for the lines or curves to dominate, they should fill most of the slide. You may need to break the x or y axis (indicated by two short parallel lines across the axis with a gap between them) in order to avoid the data appearing only at the top or right of the graph.

▲ Be consistent with tick marks

Tick marks (the little lines that indicate values on the x and y axes) should be either 'in' or 'out', and should be consistent on all your slides. Generally speaking, 'out' works better on slides, and the tick marks are then distinct from the lines on the graph.

▲ Don't forget that you can add extra information to amplify what you're saying

Provided you don't clutter up the graph with too much extra information, you can enhance audience understanding by highlighting key points on your line graphs. For example, if you are showing changes in a hormone level over time you might like to include a horizontal line to indicate a normal level, or you might like to indicate the point at which two lines start to diverge.

17

Slide preparation: bar charts

Bar charts are widely used to present data in scientific presentations. Follow these simple tips to use them effectively and appropriately.

▲ Use bar charts where the independent variable is discontinuous

Use bar charts where the independent variable (the x axis) is discontinuous – for example, you might be comparing the effects of two different treatments on a single outcome in three different patient groups. Treatment effect (the continuous dependent variable) would be measured on the y axis, and so there would be three sets of paired bars.

▲ Have no more than seven bars on a graph

You should have no more than seven bars on a graph, unless the bars are paired, in which case up to five pairs are permissible.

▲ Avoid three-dimensional bar graphs

Three-dimensional bar graphs may look attractive at first sight, but we would advise avoiding them – statisticians hate them, and it is more or less impossible to add error bars to them. Two-dimensional bar charts are fine. If you really feel the need to give the illusion of a solid structure, try the shading feature in PowerPoint that makes bars look as though they are slightly rounded, but does not actually make them three-dimensional. (Click on the bars, select 'Format data series', then 'Fill effects'.)

▲ Add selected *P* values

If you are making statistical comparisons between bars, you can include *P* values on the graph, using lines to indicate which bars are being compared. However, you may need to select which comparisons to show, or you could end up with a messy chart.

▲ Very simple bar charts are acceptable …

In a paper, most journals are reluctant to accept bar charts with just two or three bars, even though this might be a nice visual way of comparing two values. In a presentation, however, there are no such restrictions. Go ahead and use a simple bar chart if you think it makes the point clearly.

▲ … But avoid presentations that consist of endless bar charts

Too much of any kind of graph can pall after a while. You may need to think about some alternative ways of presenting the data.

▲ You can use horizontal bar charts if the labels are too long to fit on the *x* axis …

For some types of bar chart, horizontal bars are more efficient – i.e. with the *x* axis vertical and the *y* axis horizontal. This might work if, for example, you were giving numbers of patients with a particular diagnosis, and the names of the conditions would be too long to fit comfortably on a horizontal *x* axis.

▲ … But don't display the same type of data in two different formats

Don't, however, use horizontal bar charts just for variety – it is confusing for the audience if the same type of data is displayed in two different ways during the presentation.

▲ Use negative bar charts for negative scales

If your data consists of negative values – for example, if you want to indicate a reduction in a particular parameter – remember that you can construct a bar chart with the *x* axis at the top instead of the bottom of the graph.

▲ Remember that you can subdivide bars

If it's relevant to your data, you can subdivide bars horizontally to show subgroups within a single group (for example, men and women). You can use tints of a single colour to indicate the different groups.

▲ If you subdivide bars, put the darkest colour at the bottom

In bars that are subdivided horizontally, the darkest tint should be at the bottom, or an optical illusion will make the bar look 'top-heavy'.

18

Slide preparation:
pie charts

▲ Pie charts show subdivisions within a single dataset

Pie charts may be used, for example, to show the proportions of different age groups within a single population, or the number of respondents to a questionnaire who answered 'yes', 'no' and 'don't know'.

▲ Have no more than seven slices in your pie

Generally speaking, pie charts become hard to understand when there are more than about seven slices in the pie. If you have too many, you could consider combining some of the smaller values as 'other'.

▲ For emphasis, cut a slice or use colour

To emphasise a particular value, you can cut a slice out of the pie using PowerPoint's pie chart functions, or use a strong colour.

▲ Start at 12 o'clock

It's usual to arrange your slices in a logical order, starting at the top of the chart (12 o'clock) and working clockwise. What constitutes a logical order depends on your data – the important thing is that it should not be random.

▲ Prefer labels to a key

A key requires too much effort from the audience, so it's preferable to label the different slices instead.

▲ Put labels on the outside of the pie

Usually, text labels are too large to fit neatly inside all the slices of the pie, so put them on the outside, arranged next to the relevant slice.

▲ Percentages are optional

If you think it would be useful for the audience, you can give percentages actually on the graph – they can go next to the labels, or if the slices are big enough, they can go within the slices with the data labels on the outside.

▲ Remember that you can break down slices with a linked pie or 100% bar

If you want to show subcategories within a single category, PowerPoint allows you to pull out a single slice of the pie, and show it broken down further into another pie or a 100% bar (which is simply a pie chart sliced in a different way).

▲ Consider 100% bars for showing more than one dataset on the same slide

You can show two pie charts on the same slide, but if you want to show more than two, 100% bars (like a rectangular cake sliced horizontally instead of radially) can show up to five datasets on the same slide.

19

Slide preparation: line drawings

Flow charts and diagrams are both examples of line drawings. PowerPoint allows you to construct flow charts automatically, and also provides various drawing tools.

▲ Use flow charts to show processes or hierarchies

Flow charts can be used to show processes (e.g. the clotting cascade) or hierarchies (e.g. taxonomic divisions of living organisms).

▲ Edit the text inside the boxes ruthlessly

Try to minimise the numbers of words inside the boxes – this will give the audience less work to do, and makes it easier to fit all the information you need into the space available.

▲ Try not to over-complicate flow charts

It may be necessary to miss out stages or to break down flow charts into several slides in order to provide the audience with a message they can easily assimilate from a single slide. For example, you could not possibly hope to get the whole of the Krebs cycle on a single slide.

▲ Use builds to make complex flow charts easier to understand

Complicated flow charts can be made easier to understand by using the 'build' technique and adding stages in the process one at a time.

▲ Flow charts can combine text and pictures

Some topics lend themselves to 'pictorial' flow charts – for example, the life cycle of a parasite, or the attachment of a virus to a host cell.

▲ Simple line drawings or flow charts can often be used to make study design clear

Where appropriate, simple line diagrams are a useful way of showing the design of a study – particularly useful, for example, for clinical trials that involve run-in periods or crossover designs.

▲ You can also express simple ideas as diagrams

It's possible to show linked ideas in diagrammatic form. This often provides welcome visual relief when the presentation would otherwise consist mainly of text slides.

▲ Line drawings can sometimes be clearer than photographs

Line drawings are often clearer than photographs – for example, if you are trying to show an anatomical feature, the construction of a piece of equipment, or a surgical procedure.

▲ Be aware of copyright issues

If you construct a new illustration based on someone else's data, always acknowledge the original source. Be aware that scanning in illustrations from other people's books and papers can potentially breach copyright. Educational users should check the rules with their University library. It may be permissible to copy material for educational purposes, but again you should acknowledge the original source on the slide. If you are using someone else's illustration for commercial purposes, you must have permission from the owner, as well as acknowledging the source. Usually, the copyright to papers is held by the journal, so you should write to them for permission; they will almost certainly request that you also write as a courtesy to the author of the paper.

20

Slide preparation: photos

▲ Photos must be of good quality in order to project successfully

If a picture is blurry in the original, imagine how it will look when projected at a much higher magnification. You can lose resolution when scanning photos, so the ideal is to use digital photographs wherever possible to avoid loss of quality.

▲ Don't show pictures of people without their permission

If someone can be identified from a photograph (e.g. a patient), you should always have their written permission to use it. It's not necessary to obtain permission to use photos of isolated body parts, however.

▲ Mask names on radiographs and other patient charts

If a patient's name appears on a radiograph, EEG, ECG, etc., you should mask it – again, it's part of your duty of patient confidentiality.

▲ Don't scan in photos without considering copyright issues

It is tempting to scan in photos from books or papers, but remember to think about copyright issues (see p. 88).

▲ Consider indicating points of interest with arrows

If you plan to point to something on a photograph during your presentation, consider whether it would be more appropriate to use a laser pointer, or whether you could save yourself some trouble by simply adding an arrow to point to the feature you want to emphasise, thus saving yourself the trouble of trying to hold the laser pointer steady.

▲ Photos often look better if they fill the entire slide

Often it is better to skip the title on a photographic slide and let the photo fill the whole screen.

21

Using flipcharts, whiteboards and blackboards effectively

The flipchart is one of the oldest visual aids, yet can still be highly effective. It is suitable for small groups (up to about 30 people). Most of the tips given here for flipcharts can also be applied to whiteboards and blackboards.

▲ Use flipcharts when you want to be (or appear to be) spontaneous

Flipcharts can help you to appear spontaneous (even if you have fully prepared what you are going to say in advance). If you are using another medium for your main presentation, flipcharts help you to give your audience something 'extra', for example to answer questions or summarise action points.

▲ Use flipcharts to vary the pace and style of the presentation

If you have a number of messages to deliver, their memorability can be enhanced by using a number of different media and by switching pace from the more formal 'PowerPoint' presentation to explaining something on the flipchart.

▲ Involve workshop participants in flipchart creation

Not only are flipcharts an ideal way to capture key points in group discussion, they offer you the chance to take a break and hand over the task of flipchart recording to workshop participants. For example, you can ask participants to summarise the outcomes of group discussions.

▲ Practise writing in large clear letters

Make sure that what you are writing is visible from the back of the room by writing in large letters, but avoid writing all in capitals, which are difficult to read. It's a good idea to practise writing on flipcharts, as it is a very different experience from writing on paper on a horizontal surface.

▲ Use strong lines

Use felt-tip markers in blue, black or green – red can be used for highlighting. Pick broad-tipped markers that stand out well.

▲ Be colourful

Vary the colour of your flipchart pens to add to the impact of your presentation. Choose colours according to some kind of logical scheme – for example, change colours as you change topics. If you are drawing graphs freehand, use different colours for the axes and the lines or bars, and use the full page of the flipchart.

▲ Consider using at least some pre-prepared flipcharts

Sometimes it is a good idea to have prepared your flipcharts in advance. This has the advantage that you can spend more time on making them look good, as you do not have the audience watching you write. To help you find your place, you can attach tabs to the prepared pages.

▲ Use an 'invisible outline'

If you want to appear spontaneous, but are afraid of missing key points, you can 'cheat' by preparing some of your flipchart pages in advance using light pencil writing, which will be visible to you but not to the audience.

▲ Think twice about using flipcharts if your spelling is really bad

You can be a great scientist but a poor speller. Nowadays, the spellcheck on your computer helps you to get things right when you are preparing PowerPoint slides, but it won't help you when you write on a flipchart. Your credibility can be undermined by poor spelling, especially if you are not well known to your audience.

▲ Don't talk and write at the same time

Under the pressure of time, you may be tempted to write on the flipchart and talk at the same time. This can be very difficult for your audience, especially if they are also trying to take notes. The rule is, tell them what you are going to tell them, write it on the flipchart, then tell them what you told them, then ask for questions or check for understanding. That way they get three bites at the cherry and your message is reinforced.

▲ Don't talk with your back to the audience

Whatever you do, do not talk while your back is turned towards the audience. Wait until you have finished writing and can turn to the audience, point to the flipchart and speak.

▲ Stick it on the wall

If your presentation is for teaching purposes, you may want to tear off some of the flipchart pages and attach them to the walls. This can reinforce key messages, and can be referred back to later in the presentation. Some flipcharts have a re-usable adhesive backing strip. Some training rooms have special strips on the wall into which you can insert flipchart sheets. Alternatively, use a 'Blu-tack'-type product – try to avoid using sticky tape, which can damage some surfaces.

22

Using the overhead projector

The overhead projector (OHP) has fallen out of favour somewhat since the widespread use of computer-generated presentations. However, despite the perception of the OHP as an 'old-fashioned' medium, it remains a flexible and effective means of supporting a presentation.

▲ Use the OHP when computer-generated or 35 mm slide presentation would be impossible or unreliable

Poorer institutions in some countries may still be using the OHP as their main means of presentation – check out what facilities are available before you turn up clutching just your laptop, compact disc (CD) or floppy disk. Many presenters also like to travel with their presentation printed out on OHP slides as a backup in case of irretrievable computer or projector breakdown. (As an alternative, you could carry a disk or hard copy from which you could print out or photocopy OHP slides in an emergency.)

▲ Consider using the OHP in informal presentations

The OHP tends to create an informal feel. It can be used as the sole means of presentation, or as an 'extra' – for example, to show answers to questions, or capture ideas and opinions from a group, in much the same way as you would use a flipchart, whiteboard or blackboard.

▲ Consider using the OHP in small groups

Like flipcharts, the OHP is best used in small groups (up to a maximum of about 30 people). It is unsuited to large conference halls, as it is impossible to project a bright, clear image at an adequate size.

▲ Use handwritten OHP slides sparingly

As we've said, you can handwrite OHP slides on the spot, to answer questions or capture your audience's ideas, but an entire presentation consisting of handwritten slides (the kind a few of us may remember from our schooldays) looks unprofessional in a modern environment, and is hard for the audience to read.

▲ When you do write by hand, write in large, clear letters

If you handwrite a slide, make sure you write in big, legible letters. Avoid using all capitals in a mistaken attempt to aid clarity – they're actually harder to read than sentence case and, as with emails, it looks as though you're shouting.

▲ Prepare slides in advance using PowerPoint or a word-processing program

In most cases, unless you are extremely confident in being (or appearing to be) spontaneous, you will probably want to prepare your slides ahead of time. You can prepare simple slides with Word or another word-processing program, but Power-Point makes it easy to create more professional-looking slides with a minimum of effort.

▲ Make sure your text will fit on the OHP projection area

European OHP projectors usually have an A4 projection area, but US projectors may have a projection area 10 inches square. To be on the safe side, use a landscape format. If you use PowerPoint and print onto A4 sheets, the PowerPoint template will normally ensure that your text fits into a 'safe' area.

▲ In general, follow the principles for PowerPoint slides

You won't go far wrong in preparing OHP slides if you follow the general principles for PowerPoint in Chapter 11. In particular:

Use a large sans serif font

A sans serif font such as Helvetica is easier to read than a serif font such as Times New Roman. It should be at least 24-point when printed out on an A4 slide – bigger is better.

Limit yourself to no more than seven bullet points per slide

No more than seven bullet points per slide (with no more than seven words in each) should be the rule – and there's nothing wrong with having fewer. Avoid the temptation to cram as much as possible onto each slide.

▲ Don't use the OHP as an opportunity to be lazy

Don't make a habit of photocopying A4 pages from textbooks onto slides – it looks dreadful and is impossible for your audience to read. There are special OHPs that allow you project directly from a printed page as well as from slides – but please use this function selectively and not as a substitute for adequate preparation.

▲ Make your slides colourful

Colour makes things stand out and is visually appealing. Colour makes it possible to highlight your key messages, enabling your audience to retain more of what you say, almost without realising it. Colour transparencies are expensive and time-consuming to print, so make sure you proofread your slides carefully before you start printing!

▲ Make it visual

As with PowerPoint slides, the more visual the presentation, the better. Try to avoid having endless text-only OHP slides – graphs, tables and even photographs work well with the OHP.

▲ Tear off paper backings before you start

It's irritating to watch presenters who pick up each slide and tear off the paper backing. It breaks the flow of the presentation, and the presenter is usually at a loss to know what to do with the mounting pile of waste paper. Make sure all your slides are ready to present before you start (you should have been rehearsing with them anyway!).

▲ Consider using frames

Frames stop excess light from 'leaking' around the edges of the slide – this excess light otherwise 'draws' the audience's eyes and is tiring to look at. 'Flip frames' (clear plastic sleeves with fold-out opaque flaps) give a professional look, especially as they line up precisely on the projector if placed against the little guideposts present on many projectors (sometimes these guideposts need to be released before use). Flip frames are easy to store in ring binders. Cardboard frames are also available, notched to line up with the guideposts on the projector. Slides in cardboard frames are more cumbersome to store than flip frames, but do have the advantage that you can write notes to yourself on the frame.

▲ Check that there is a replacement bulb and that you know how to change it

The OHP is a very robust piece of equipment – the most common problem is simply a burnt-out bulb. Most have a spare bulb already in place, so that you can simply switch over when a bulb blows. But make sure that there is actually a spare installed and that you know where the switch is, so that you don't get flustered in the middle of your presentation.

▲ Stand on the 'correct' side of the projector

If you are right-handed, the OHP should be on your right as you face the audience. If you are left-handed, the projector should be on your left. That way, you will find changing the slides less awkward.

▲ Put your pointer on the projector instead of pointing at the screen

One advantage of the OHP is that you don't need to turn your back to the audience to point at the screen. Instead, you can use a pen or pencil as a pointer, placing it directly on the slide, and leaving it there as long as you are emphasising or explaining the point to the audience.

▲ Face your audience

As with any other kind of presentation, look at your audience and avoid turning round to look at the screen. This should be easy to do because the slides are on the OHP in front of you.

▲ Avoid the 'striptease' effect

No doubt we have all seen presentations where the presenter masks the slide with a piece of paper and, as the presentation continues, the paper is tantalisingly slid down further and further to reveal successive points. Usually it gets to about the halfway point when the breeze from the projector's fan or gravity intervenes, and the paper falls to the floor. If you don't want your audience to see consecutive points before you are ready to present them, consider putting them onto successive separate slides. If you must use the 'striptease' routine, put the paper mask *under* the slide and then it won't fall off halfway through.

▲ Don't read the slide

Try to avoid reading the slide as if it were your notes. The audience is quite capable of reading it too and is looking for more explanation from you. The text or image should support what you are saying. Try to look at the audience, and maintain eye contact – the slide will still be there as backup if you lose the thread of what you are saying.

▲ Think about whether to switch off the projector when changing slides

Some presenters believe that you should always switch off the projector when changing slides. In theory, this avoids annoying the audience by showing them a brightly lit blank screen. However, it can be very irritating (to you and the audience) if you are moving through the slides quickly. Some projectors have a switch that allows the lamp to be switched off independently of the fan, which helps. Whether or not you decide to turn off the lamp between slides, remember to turn it off during the discussion.

▲ Take an 'OHP survival kit' with you

Depending on the circumstances, an 'OHP survival kit' might contain:

- extension cord
- adaptor plugs (depending on country)
- spare bulb
- OHP pens
- spare OHP transparencies.

23

Using video effectively

It is unlikely that you would use video for the whole of your presentation (after all, what would be the point of your being there?), but it can be a very powerful and engaging tool for occasional use during your talk.

▲ Make sure your video is relevant

Using video purely for novelty value is likely to backfire. Make sure the content adds something to your scientific story, supports your argument, and does not dominate the whole presentation.

▲ Videos can be home-made …

Typical examples of 'home-made' videos include recordings of investigations, procedures or experiments. Clinicians can also use recordings of patient interviews or consultations, for which you will need the patient's written permission.

▲ … Or bought from commercial sources

Depending on your subject matter, you may also be able to find relevant videos that have been commercially prepared for teaching purposes. These can be used to add variety to your presentation.

▲ Remember that TV programmes are copyrighted

Sometimes you will see something relevant as part of a science programme on TV. Remember, however, that programmes are copyrighted. You cannot show clips from them without permission, which may require the payment of a fee. Many TV companies have special arrangements for educational institutions to obtain copies of scientific documentaries, and a scale of charges.

▲ Keep your video clips short …

Bear in mind that, for maximum impact, video clips within a conference presentation should be kept short – ideally no more than one or two minutes. Why? Because after a couple of minutes of watching a video, the audience begins to forget about you as the presenter. They begin to settle down comfortably to 'watch the movie'. However, in a conference presentation, you want to keep the audience alert and focused on you and your data.

▲ … Unless the video can be considered as a presentation in itself

Sometimes, the video itself is the presentation, and the presenter takes a back seat. For example, videos are often used in a training situation, where trainers use the video to give the participants a change of pace, and to actually take away attention from them as the presenter.

▲ Think carefully about how many video clips you use

The audience has come to see you, not watch a movie. Except in special circumstances, one or two video clips per presentation are usually enough.

▲ Where possible, provide a 'live' commentary

One way of retaining the audience's focus on you during a video clip is to provide the commentary 'live' youself, rather than relying on any pre-recorded commentary.

▲ In a teaching situation, ask students to take notes

If you are in a teaching setting, ask the students to take notes from the video for later discussion. This will ensure that they remain attentive and do not use the video as an opportunity to 'tune out'.

24

Rehearsing your presentation

Even the most experienced presenters need to rehearse. Rehearsal will help you to overcome nerves, see how your presentation works in practice, iron out any potential problems with the slides, and make sure your presentation fits the allotted time.

▲ Check that you've selected the right number of slides

Having carefully prepared your slides so that they are clear and readable, you need to check that you have the correct number. There is no point in having 40 or more slides for a 20-minute presentation. Decide how much you want to say about each of the main points and then how many slides you will need to illustrate each point.

▲ Check the slides are in the right order

Check the order of the slides so that the flow is logical. With 35 mm slides, check that they are all the right way around and that none of them are broken.

▲ Check your timing by speaking out loud

If you have been asked to speak for 20 minutes, be ruthless about sticking to time. Remember that delivering your presentation at the correct speed will probably take longer than you think – a 'mental rehearsal' is always faster than the real thing. So make sure that you actually practise the whole presentation out loud, including pauses.

▲ Try practising with a tape recorder

Recording your presentation onto a tape will highlight a number of useful factors:

- How fast are you speaking?
- Are you taking enough pauses?
- Are you using different tones and emphasis?
- How expressive are you?
- Does it sound interesting to somebody else?
- Do you have any verbal 'tics' or do you 'um' and 'er' a lot?

▲ Use a mirror to check your body language …

Rehearsing in front of a mirror is a good way of checking your posture, gestures and general delivery. You can also practise gaining eye contact with your own image.

▲ … Or even better, a video recording …

The video will allow you to check every aspect of your voice and body language:

- Do you look at the slide projection screen or at the audience?
- Do you have your head buried in your notes?
- Do you cling to the lectern for support?
- Do you look welcoming, or do you put up a psychological barrier between yourself and the audience?
- Do you stand confidently or hop from one foot to the other?
- Do you use the visual aids and pointer confidently?
- Do you sweep the room with your gaze, getting eye contact with the audience?

▲ … Or your friends, family or partner

If you do not have access to a video recorder, you can rehearse your presentation in front of your family or friends. Explain the purpose of the rehearsal and ask them to be as objective as possible, otherwise they may be too kind to you! Even adverse comments will help you and should not be taken as personal criticism.

▲ For important presentations, do a formal trial run

Following the preliminary rehearsal and before the big day, it is sometimes a good idea to do a trial run in a less critical, relatively safe environment. For example, you may have students or colleagues to whom you could give the presentation before delivering it at a major international meeting.

▲ Form reciprocal relationships to critique each other's presentations

You can set up reciprocal relationships with colleagues to critique each other's talks. Make sure you give each other balanced feedback – be generous with your praise, and concentrate on one point for improvement each time. Make sure you separate the behaviour from the person to avoid hurting people's feelings.

25

Keeping track

Keeping track of where you are in your presentation is important, particularly if you need to respond to a question during the talk and then return to the flow. There are several options available, which you choose is simply a matter of personal preference.

▲ A mind map allows you to see your whole talk on one sheet of paper

If you are familiar with mind mapping (see p. 18), notes in this format are compact and very easy to follow. Unlike linear, sequential notes, mind mapping involves displaying all the major points as an array on a single piece of paper with links and subdivisions connected with lines.

▲ Use PowerPoint notes or handout pages to match your slides

If you have produced your slides as a PowerPoint presentation, you can print out a hard copy of the notes pages, which will have a picture of each slide and a space below for text. This can be useful for tracking exactly what you wanted to say about each individual slide. Alternatively you may just want to print out the handout pages, which show a miniature version of each slide, with three or six slides per page. Number the pages of your notes, or staple them together at one corner, in case you drop them or get them mixed up.

▲ Use file cards if you find them easier to handle than sheets of A4 paper

File cards such as those used for addresses are a neat and unobtrusive way of keeping notes. As with notes pages, file cards should always be numbered. One card per slide is a good way to keep track.

▲ Use a written script/it makes you feel more secure

If you have written a script for your presentation, even though you do not intend to read from it, it can offer the ultimate security backup. Highlight the main points with a coloured pen so that they are easy to pick out during delivery of the presentation, as your eye will be drawn to the highlighted sections. Add slide numbers in the margin.

▲ Make sure any written notes or file cards are legible

- Always use large type or handwriting to make your notes stand out clearly.
- Make all your abbreviations clear and meaningful to you.
- Add references to slides.
- Use only one side of the page or card.
- Highlight new topics and conclusions.
- Number your notes or file cards.

▲ Keep track of time as well as content

Keeping track of time is important for both you and your audience. If you start to run over time, they will become restless and will not be listening. If you finish too early, they may feel short-changed. Add timings to your notes (e.g. halfway, here by 10.15, etc.).

▲ Make sure you can see the time easily

Look for a clock in the room (and check if it's showing the same time as your watch). If there's no clock, you could bring a small travelling clock to put on the lectern, or put your wristwatch on the lectern so you don't have to take an obvious look at your wrist (don't leave it behind when you leave the stage).

▲ Consider making use of a 'timekeeper' in the audience

You could ask a friend in the audience to be your timekeeper, so that at a pre-arranged signal you begin your summary and conclusion to your talk.

26

Arriving well prepared

There are many things to check the week before the presentation, especially if it involves some travel. Devise your own checklist, and keep it on hand for future meetings.

▲ Check the arrangements carefully

Be sure to check that you have the right date, time, place, and what sort of equipment will be available.

▲ Check travel documents and money

Do you have:

- a valid passport (with visas if needed)
- tickets
- money (you will probably need foreign currency for a taxi when you arrive)
- credit cards or traveller's cheques, PIN numbers for ATMs?

▲ Check your mobile phone

Do you know how to:

- change the band/network if necessary
- retrieve your messages?

▲ Check you have key phone numbers

Do you have phone numbers for:

- your hotel
- your airline
- the conference centre
- the conference contact person
- your credit card company?

▲ Check you know how to get to the venue

- Do you have a map of the area?
- Do you have details of how to reach the venue?
- Will you be met and if so where?

▲ Check you have the right clothes

Find out about the climate and what sort of clothing you will need – both formal and informal. If you are travelling by plane, think about whether you can manage with hand luggage only. If you must take hold baggage, make sure you either wear or carry clothes that you could present in, if the airline were to lose your luggage.

▲ Make sure you have any regular medication and remedies for common ailments

Do you need to take any special medication with you, for example:

- aspirin for preventing 'traveller's thrombosis'
- antihistamines for rhinitis or hay fever
- inhalers for asthma
- headache or migraine remedies
- diarrhoea remedies
- indigestion remedies
- travel sickness remedies
- cough and cold remedies
- throat lozenges
- beta-blockers for nerves?

▲ Make yourself comfortable

If you are flying long distance, think about other useful items to make your journey more comfortable. Earplugs can minimise background noise, helping you to sleep and arrive more refreshed. You might like to take an inflatable pillow to support your neck.

▲ Make sure you have an alarm clock

The last thing you want to do is to oversleep and be late, so pack your alarm clock, or make sure you can use the alarm function on your mobile phone, watch, personal organiser or computer. You can use the hotel's alarm call facilities as a backup. Waking up can be a particular concern if you are travelling to a different time zone.

▲ Check who will be responsible for technical matters

Find out if there is an audio-visual technician, or whether you will be in charge of setting up your own equipment on the day.

▲ If you are using 35 mm slides, do you need to take a carousel?

If you are using 35 mm slides, make sure you know what sort of projector is being used. Ascertain whether the organisers will provide a spare carousel, or whether you should take your own.

▲ If your presentation is computerised, do you need to take a laptop?

Check whether you will be using your own laptop or if a computer is provided. If you are using someone else's computer, how should you provide your slides:

- emailed in advance
- on a floppy disk
- on a CD
- on a portable universal serial bus (USB) drive?

▲ If you are using someone else's computer, check software compatibility

You should check the compatibility of your slide presentation software, for example that the presentation can be unzipped (if it is a large file with lots of graphics) or that the laptop has a floppy drive or CD ROM drive. If you are running the presentation from your hard disk, make sure you have a backup available (e.g. floppy disk, CD, or USB drive).

▲ Check and recheck your equipment

Try out every piece of equipment you plan to use, making sure that it works (and that you know how to work it).

▲ Check your power supply

Make sure you have all the batteries, cables and adaptors you need. Take spare batteries with you for items like remote controls and laser pointers.

▲ Check you have all the materials needed for an interactive seminar

If your presentation is an interactive seminar and participants are involved in group work, make sure you have all the necessary equipment such as flipcharts with replacement paper, marker pens, OHP acetates, 'Blu-tack', pins, scissors and sticky tape.

▲ Check audiotapes, videos and digital video disks (DVDs)

Check that any videotapes or DVDs you wish to show are compatible with the equipment available, as systems differ between Europe and the US. Cue audio and videotapes to exactly the right point. If you are using CDs or minidisks to play music or a soundtrack, make sure you know how to make them start in the right place.

27

Last-minute checks

The big day has arrived and you have prepared thoroughly. Here are a few last-minute points to ensure complete success.

▲ In unfamiliar countries, be thoughtful about what you eat and drink

Depending on the country and your own constitution, you should avoid any foods commonly associated with stomach upsets, such as shellfish, unpeeled fruit and vegetables and tap water (including ice in drinks). Try to avoid foods that may be considered antisocial, like strong onions or garlic. To ensure that you feel as lively as possible on the day of the presentation, avoid alcohol the night before and drink plenty of water (bottled if necessary).

▲ Arrive early

Make sure you arrive early, in plenty of time for your presentation. Always assume that the taxi will take twice as long as people tell you and that the traffic will be the worst ever.

▲ If you can, check your slides one last time

If you are presenting at a major congress, there is often a preview room for speakers. Sometimes there may be a sponsor who is handling the arrangements and will be keen to help with your slides.

▲ Check the equipment and who will be operating it

Ensure that you are familiar with the equipment and with who does what. For example, with computerised slides, will you start your own slides or will a technician? With 35 mm slides, who is responsible for loading and unloading the slides?

▲ Make sure you meet and greet all necessary officials

If you are part of a bigger meeting, take the time to meet the chairperson and the other speakers. There may be simultaneous translation, in which case the interpreters will want a copy of your notes and will want to hear you speak before the presentation.

▲ Check the room layout

If you are presenting at a large congress, take the time to visit the room and check things like layout, where you will sit before and after the presentation, how you get up on to the stage, and the position of the lectern, so that there are no surprises on the day.

▲ Check the equipment

35 mm slides

Check the focus and that you are familiar with operating the remote control, including going backwards as well as forwards. Check that there is a spare bulb and whether back or front projection is used.

OHP presentation

Check that there is a spare bulb and that the OHP is properly set up with the cables safely taped down. Check the focus of the OHP, and that the slides fill the screen and can be seen from anywhere in the room. Ideally the screen should tilt forward slightly at the top to avoid any parallax distortion. Make sure there is a table nearby for your notes and OHP slides.

Computerised presentation

Check the mouse, remote or conventional. If there is no technical support available, check that you know how to connect any necessary cables to the data projector, how to turn it on, off and to standby, and how to switch to the right input. If you are using your own laptop, try to make sure that it works with the data projector – it will probably need to load new drivers. If you are using an old data projector with a new laptop, and it doesn't work at first, try changing to a lower monitor resolution on the laptop – sometimes high resolution is incompatible with older projectors.

Other electrical items

Make sure you have sufficient sockets or a plug board for all the equipment. If you are using video, familiarise yourself with the operation of the TV and video cassette recorder (VCR).

Your microphone

If you are using a microphone, there is usually a technician available to set the equipment up. If you've never used a microphone before, ask if you can practise prior to your presentation. This will boost your confidence and remove any uncertainty before the big day.

▲ Check your personal bits and pieces

Check that you have your watch or clock for timekeeping, your notes, a drink of water, throat lozenges (if you use them) and any lucky charms or mascots.

28

Delivering your presentation: basic principles

Now you have prepared your presentation, it's time to deliver it. Here are some simple tips to help make it more of a pleasure than an ordeal.

▲ Be well prepared

If you arrive flustered, or if you find halfway through the presentation that your slides do not match what you want to say, you're unlikely to be able to deliver the presentation effectively. So check, check and check again – slides, equipment, notes, venue, time, etc.

▲ Practise – and then practise again

Rehearse your presentation thoroughly. If possible, have a 'trial run' in front of an audience of sympathetic colleagues, so that you can also practise responding to questions.

▲ Be enthusiastic – or fake it

Even if you are not particularly happy to be giving the presentation, or if you have talked about this topic many times before, do your best to act as if you are enthusiastic – at least for the duration of the presentation. Your enthusiasm will be infectious, and audiences are more disposed to forgive minor slips if it is obvious that you really enjoy your topic.

▲ Seek feedback

The more presentations you give, the better you will perform – provided you have some way of knowing how you are doing. So be open to feedback, even if it is uncomfortable. Try to have a friendly colleague in the audience who will give you constructive criticism afterwards. In teaching situations, students will often be invited to complete feedback forms – try not to take any adverse comments personally, but learn from them for future occasions.

▲ Be flexible

Presentations don't always go exactly according to plan, however carefully you have prepared. That's one reason why it would be wrong to learn your presentation word-for-word and deliver it like a tape-recorder. Be flexible, so that if things do not go exactly to plan you can adapt to meet the new situation.

▲ Be adventurous – but try it out first

It's good to be open to new ways of presenting the same data, or to changes in your personal style, but make sure you try out new ideas in a safe environment where you can obtain honest feedback – a major presentation at an international meeting is not the place to try out your video clips or a new anecdote for the first time.

▲ Focus on the 'three Rs'

Focusing on the 'three Rs' – *rapport, relevance* and *richness* – will help you to deliver a powerful presentation. What we mean by this is detailed in the three tips below.

Establish rapport with your audience

Rapport is the feeling of connection that you, as a speaker, have with the audience. It comes from really understanding the audience's needs and being able to put yourself in their shoes. Rapport can be developed by asking yourself:

- Why have I been asked to speak?
- What special knowledge or viewpoint do I have?
- Why is my subject important to me?
- What kind of presenter do I aspire to be?

Expressing empathy with the audience will get them on your side straight away and they will warm to you and your theme. The opposite approach is to be aloof and arrogant, in which case the audience will be eagerly awaiting your failure.

Make your presentation relevant

During the preparation of your presentation you will have considered questions like:

- What is the purpose of my presentation?
- What will be most interesting to my audience?
- What is my message?
- Which three concepts are most important?
- What actions do I expect my audience to take?

Mentally reviewing these points will ensure that you are in the right frame of mind to make the presentation truly relevant to the audience.

Make your presentation 'rich'

Richness in a presentation comes from invoking as many of the audience's senses as possible. We all experience things in a different and unique way. We have different preferences for how we like to absorb information, via three possible routes:

- visual (i.e. the slides or other visual aids)
- auditory (i.e. the talk)
- kinaesthetic (i.e. physical experience).

Most people can learn through all three routes, but we also have a dominant route. Visual people have a preference for seeing information, e.g. slides, flipcharts or videos. Auditory people prefer the spoken (and written) word, e.g. talks, tapes or radio programmes. Kinaesthetic people are 'hands-on' and need to experience what they are hearing about, e.g. through group exercises or demonstrations. Ideally, your presentation should contain elements that satisfy all three types of people.

Add visual richness

Visual richness starts with the selection of visual aids and the choice of images and colours for your slides. But it also extends to you – you are, in fact, the most important visual aid. How you stand, how you use your body and how you use gestures are all-important.

Add auditory richness

Auditory richness includes how you use your voice, the audibility, articulation, and appropriateness of what you are saying, as well as the language you use.

Add kinaesthetic richness

Kinaesthetic richness depends on your motion and emotion and your audience's motion and emotion. Your movements and gestures should demonstrate high levels of energy. Consider how close you wish to stand to the audience, and whether you want to walk amongst them or give out a handout. Your emotion will be conveyed by the belief you have in your ideas, the genuine pleasure you derive from communicating, showing the audience why you care, and the difference it makes to you. In informal situations, you can also engage your audience kinaesthetically by asking for a show of hands, asking them questions, using demonstrations or breaking them into groups for short exercises. If they have been sitting for a long period, you could even get them to stand up and stretch or walk around. Asking questions of the audience, quoting wise or learned people, or telling anecdotes will also increase emotional involvement and add to the richness of the presentation.

▲ Involving people in your presentations can add interest

Sometimes it is useful and fun to give a live demonstration using a volunteer from the audience, e.g. to illustrate some aspect of human ability or behaviour. Clinical presentations can interview or examine real patients (within ethical boundaries, of course). Sometimes a video is more manageable and more ethical than a live person – the human element still adds interest.

▲ Use props, where relevant

Props can be effective, but should have a clear purpose. Props might include pieces of technical equipment, or a distinctive timer for timing breakout sessions. With all props, make sure you are well prepared or the demonstration will spoil your presentation instead of enhancing it.

▲ Consider using music before your presentation and during breaks

Music can also be an effective way of calming or energising the audience before a presentation, or of indicating a break between sessions. Since people can have strong feelings about music, it's safest to stick to familiar classical pieces or the rather bland but inoffensive tapes specially produced for conferences.

▲ Practise physically handling your equipment

Before starting the presentation you will have already familiarised yourself with the equipment (OHP, slide projector, laptop, etc). Make sure all the controls are within easy reach, especially any remote controls and pointers.

▲ Avoid having both hands full

Try to avoid the 'full hand syndrome' with a remote control in one hand and a pointer in the other.

▲ Don't talk with your back to the audience when using a pointer

If you are pointing something out on the screen, the rule is turn, point, turn to the audience and talk. Don't talk with your back to the audience.

▲ Don't keep laser pointers on all the time

When you use a laser pointer, highlight the area of interest and then switch the pointer off. It is extremely distracting to see the red dot dance all over the screen and up the wall. If you are not actively using the pointer, put it down to discourage you from fiddling with it.

▲ With OHP acetates, put the pointer on the OHP

If you're using an OHP, leave the pointer on the acetate, rather than pointing at the screen.

29

Delivering your presentation: your voice

Your voice is one of the things that make you a unique and memorable presenter. You can't radically change the voice you grew up with, but you can practise using it at its best during the presentation.

▲ Choose your language to suit the audience

As described in 'Choosing and using words' (Chapter 9), use short, simple words for everyday things. You will, of course, need to use some long scientific words, but there's no reason why the rest of your language should be complicated. If you use long, difficult words the audience will not be impressed and half of them may be distracted while they puzzle over what you are saying.

▲ Don't speak too fast

Your voice is a powerful medium, and how you use it can affect the way the audience responds. The speed at which you speak will depend on the language capability of the audience. For non-native speakers, you will need to speak more slowly; in small groups, you can ask for audience feedback on the speed. We generally speak too quickly – what seems like slow speech to us when presenting is a normal speed for the audience.

▲ Vary the speed at which you speak

Try varying the pace and watch the effects it has on the audience. Occasional deliberate increases in pace can have an energising effect on the audience.

▲ Practise a friendly, confident tone

You should adopt a friendly, confident tone that is inviting to listen to, and not too authoritative or aloof. Sometimes it helps to imagine you are talking to just one person. Vary your expression and emotion for effect. Try saying 'a million pounds' quickly as if it was a trivial sum and the answer to the question 'What's 500 thousand pounds plus 500 thousand pounds?' Now say '50 thousand pounds' slowly with feeling, as if it were a huge sum of money. Which one sounds more?

▲ Check the volume of your voice

Make sure you can be heard by the person at the back of the room – especially if you are not using a microphone. You can vary the volume of your voice to emphasise a point or to re-energise a flagging audience.

▲ Avoid things that increase the pitch of your voice

A high-pitched, squeaky voice is tiring to listen to, as is an excessively low-pitched, croaky voice. Although there is little we can do about our voice's natural pitch, we can make the best of what we have. Avoiding overindulgence in alcohol and tobacco the night before will ensure that you are not croaking like a frog the next morning. Deep breathing just before you present will open up the vocal chords and help with controlling any nerves. Some presenters like to gargle with mouthwash, suck lozenges or even sing before they go on.

▲ Take regular pauses

Pauses are a very important part of delivery. You need to allow time for people to consider what you've said, especially after making a major point or asking a rhetorical question. As you move onto a new topic, signpost it with a bridging word or phrase like 'So how does this affect our understanding of ...?', or 'You may be wondering what this has got to do with ...' Then pause for a count of two seconds. It will convey weight and get the audience leaning forward attentively. If you have asked the audience a question, pause to allow sufficient time for them to consider it; don't be tempted to rush in too quickly.

▲ Pause after changing each slide

It is a good idea to pause after changing each visual for two seconds (count one thousand elephants, two thousand elephants). This gives the audience time to take in the slide before you start to explain it.

▲ Take more pauses if your talk is being translated

If your talk is being simultaneously translated you will need to take regular small pauses to allow for the translator to catch up.

▲ Practise using a microphone

If you have not used a microphone before, try and get some practice before your presentation. Hearing your own voice through a public address system can be quite disconcerting the first time. Tie or lapel microphones are preferred, as they do not restrict movement. A lectern microphone anchors you to the spot and you need to be aware of volume changes as you look up at the audience or to each side.

30

Delivering your presentation: body language

Studies in psychology suggest that body language accounts for about half of all communication. So, even in formal situations, it's not just what you say that counts, or even your voice. What you do with your body during the presentation can make all the difference to the way the audience perceives you, and the credibility of your message.

▲ Practise a confident stance

To project confidence, stand with your feet shoulder-width apart, head up and hands loosely by your sides, with the palms facing outwards. Your jacket should be buttoned (unless it is so tight that it rides up when you move your arms). This feels a little strange at first, but reliably conveys a message of openness and ease.

▲ Avoid defensive or tense postures

Standing with folded arms or holding your hands together in front of your body looks defensive (even if you're doing it because you feel cold). If you are standing at a lectern, avoid gripping the sides of it as if for support.

▲ Plan what you are going to do with your hands

If you have trouble standing with your hands loosely by your sides (except when you are making gestures), you could try resting one of them lightly on the lectern. It may be tempting to put your hands in your pockets to try to appear relaxed, but in fact it looks excessively casual, and may be considered downright disrespectful in some countries. Clasping your hands together behind your back may stop you from fidgeting, but looks unnatural and tense.

▲ Stand centre-stage, if you can

The preferred position is centre-stage, though this is not always possible depending on the position of the screen.

▲ Use a lectern in formal situations ...

A lectern has the advantage of giving you somewhere to put your notes, or your laptop. Some may incorporate a fixed microphone, or a computer display showing you what is on the screen behind you. So, it's appropriate to use a lectern in formal presentations in which you will need to make use of these features.

▲ ... But remember that a lectern limits communication

The disadvantage of standing at a lectern is that it limits your use of body language, thus preventing you from adding kinaesthetic richness to your presentation. So, in informal situations, it's better to dispense with the lectern and give yourself the freedom to move around the stage, or among the seminar participants.

▲ Make all movement purposeful

Movement is good, but it must be purposeful. Many presenters wander around the stage aimlessly, or rock backwards and forwards. This is distracting for the audience and reflects a lack of confidence. If the setting allows, walking towards the audience conveys interest, especially if someone has just asked a question.

▲ Practise a few gestures to emphasise important points

Even formal presentations from behind a lectern can be enhanced by a few dramatic arm and hand gestures. Pick a few key points in your presentation that you can emphasise with a gesture. Practise your gestures in front of a mirror, then try them out on a live audience in a 'safe' environment.

▲ Make your gestures large

Gestures should be expansive and made from the shoulder, not the elbow. What may seem like an exaggerated movement to you will look natural to the audience. Try to make all movement from above the waist. Make sure gestures are for emphasis and not just at random, and that your hands are clearly visible.

▲ Mirror the body language you want to see

If you want your audience to appear welcoming and friendly, then you have to appear welcoming and friendly to them first. You need to mirror the response you want to see from your audience. Smile at them and they will smile back at you – it's very hard to resist. Give out what you want to receive, and act as a good example to your audience.

▲ Show appropriate emotion in your facial expression

Make sure your body language is congruent with your message. Smiling in welcome is fine, but smiling when you are talking about a fatal disease is not.

▲ Make eye contact …

Before you even start to speak, make eye contact with one or two of the audience. This will engage them and signal to all that you are ready to begin. Try and spread the eye contact around the group, not missing any section out. You can use eye contact to invite comment from an individual, or when referring to their area of interest or expertise. This will make them feel acknowledged and valued.

▲ … Even with large audiences …

With a large audience, pick out individuals in zones and concentrate on them. The people sitting in front, behind and to the side will also feel that you are looking at them. Be a lighthouse and sweep the room with your gaze.

▲ … But be sensitive to cultural and personal differences

Note that in some countries (e.g. Japan) sustained eye contact can be considered rude or threatening. And whatever the culture, some individuals may feel uncomfortable with eye contact – if someone immediately looks away when you make eye contact, avoid looking directly into their eyes again.

▲ Watch out for audience body language

Keep an eye on the audience's body language. Look out for:

- facial expressions indicating interest, distress, enthusiasm, confusion, boredom or acceptance
- leaning forward (interest) or backward (lack of interest or tiredness)
- crossing arms or legs (resistance to your message)
- hands over mouths (stifling yawns)
- looking around the room or throat clearing (boredom)
- nodding (agreement and interest).

▲ Don't play with objects

Fiddling with pens, pointers and papers on the lectern or table in front of you is distracting, as is playing with your hair, glasses, earrings, buttons or other bits and pieces. Playing with your lapel microphone is liable to lead to unwelcome noises! In addition, try to avoid touching your face or stroking your chin.

▲ Remove temptation wherever possible

If you don't keep loose change in your pocket, you won't be able to jingle it. If you don't wear earrings, you won't be able to twiddle them.

▲ Get help in breaking irritating habits

Get a friend to watch you present, and to raise their hand every time you start to fidget. They can also help you by pointing out the verbal tics – 'ums' and 'ers' – or the repeated use of a phrase like 'all right?' or 'you know?'. Other irritating habits like throat clearing, standing in front of the screen or with your back to the audience can be identified with video or a friend's help.

▲ Write a note to yourself

If you really have a problem eradicating a habit, and you can't avoid the situation, try writing **DON'T FIDGET** in big letters on every page of your lecture notes.

31

Keeping up appearances

Your appearance affects the way that people perceive you, no matter how unfair that may be. Psychologists have found that attractive people are more persuasive than unattractive people. However, anyone can cultivate attractiveness, through good grooming and a professional approach.

▲ Be a conformist

Your audience will have certain expectations about your appearance and it is important to conform to the norm to establish and maintain rapport with them. What you choose to wear tells people about your perception of the audience and your perception of yourself.

▲ Find out what's normal

Dress norms are influenced both by national culture and by the type of meeting. At some European and North American academic meetings, many participants will wear casual clothes, whereas at big international meetings, business suits are typically worn. In the Far East, conference wear is usually very formal.

▲ Match the clothes to the setting and the audience

If you wear bright, lightweight clothes to a formal presentation you will appear lightweight, whereas if you wear a dull, sombre suit to an informal gathering you will appear dull and uninteresting.

▲ If in doubt, be too formal rather than too informal

It is a compliment to the audience that you have made the effort. Formal dress also tends to convey an air of authority or expertise. A rough rule of thumb is to aim at being 10% smarter than your audience. At international conferences this generally means a dark suit and tie for men and a business suit and blouse for women.

▲ Choose your colours with care

Dark colours are associated with power, whereas bright colours say 'look at me'. Bright colours can be memorable, and are more acceptable for women – a red jacket may help people to remember you. With smaller audiences, especially memorable clothes may outshine your message.

▲ Avoid being memorable for the wrong reasons

Large printed designs should be avoided as they are distracting to the audience. Try not to dress in an excessively trendy or overtly sexy way.

▲ Dress to suit the temperature

You need to feel comfortable to be confident in presenting. Take into account the temperature of the room – in a hot room, you can soon begin to sweat, and this makes you look flustered even if you are not.

▲ Avoid easily creased fabrics

Creased clothes that do not pack well can make you look crumpled and tired. Be especially careful about linen and silk – you may think that linen can look fashionably creased, but the less fashion-conscious members of your audience may simply think you can't be bothered to press your suit.

▲ Go for clean, conservative hairstyles

Hair that appears greasy, dirty or unkempt is off-putting to the audience. Exaggerated styles are distracting and are best avoided. Hair should be well groomed and under control.

▲ Tie long hair back or up

It is extremely distracting for an audience if the speaker is continually fiddling with his or her hair or tossing back long locks. Generally, long hair should be worn up or tied back to look businesslike and professional.

▲ Be thoughtful about facial hair

In business environments, the received wisdom is that a clean-shaven face is preferable, as this gives a message of nothing to hide. However, this is not necessarily true in scientific circles, where individuality is more respected.

▲ Don't do anything drastic to your appearance before a presentation

Avoid changing your hairstyle or colour the day before an important presentation. If you don't like it, you will feel self-conscious and it will show.

▲ Be conservative with your shoes

Shoes should be comfortable and well maintained. For women, court shoes with a medium sized heel are preferable to open-toed sandals or sexy high heels. For men, plain lace-up shoes are considered smarter than loafer-type shoes. Trainers should be avoided in all but the most informal situations.

▲ Don't wear new shoes

Never wear brand new shoes for the first time at a presentation. If they are the slightest bit tight you will be uncomfortable and self-conscious. Check that your shoes do not squeak – this will be extremely distracting for anyone sitting near you.

32

Handling presentation nerves

Practically everyone suffers from nerves to some extent before presenting. Good preparation and rehearsal will help to prevent unnecessary jitters, but some degree of tension is still natural. Here's how to minimise counterproductive nervousness, and turn the remaining state of heightened awareness to your advantage.

▲ Remember that adrenaline is not necessarily a bad thing

Some degree of nervousness is beneficial – the accompanying adrenaline surge is what puts the polish in our performance and gives us a 'high' afterwards.

▲ Learn the first few lines of your presentation by heart

It is usually a good idea to learn the first few lines of your presentation by heart so that you can concentrate on your composure as you begin to speak.

▲ Consider using beta-blockers to control shaking

If presentation nerves cause your hands to shake and your voice to wobble, your doctor may consider prescribing a beta-blocker for use on the day of the presentation. While some people benefit greatly from controlling the physical manifestations of fear in this way, it's not for everyone. There is a danger that you may come over as being too 'laid back' or 'flat', so try it out before the big day.

▲ Avoid alcohol ...

It may be tempting to try to calm yourself down with a quick drink. However, alcohol impairs your judgement of your own performance, and what may seem calm and confident to you may appear as a lacklustre or overly casual performance to the audience.

▲ ... And caffeine

Anyone sensitive to caffeine should avoid drinking excessive amounts of coffee before a presentation, as it can exacerbate shaking hands and general 'twitchiness'.

▲ Channel nervous energy into your gestures

Making expansive gestures is a useful outlet for your nervous energy, but avoid pacing up and down the stage as a result of nerves.

▲ Get some exercise before your presentation

Taking a short brisk walk before your presentation will help to stimulate deep breathing and control nerves. Alternatively you could try some isometric exercises or clenching and relaxing your fists.

▲ Try breathing or relaxation exercises

Some people find breathing or relaxation exercises helpful in controlling presentation nerves. In any case, most people find it helpful to take three long, deep, slow breaths before getting up to speak.

▲ Have water handy in case you get a dry mouth

Make sure you have some water to hand to help a dry mouth, which usually disappears after the first few sentences.

▲ Try visualisation to help you feel positive

It is sometimes helpful to imagine a situation where you were particularly successful, such as a presentation that went well. In the days leading up to your presentation, repeatedly relive the scene of your previous success in your mind, complete with the sights, sounds and feelings you felt when it all went well. Then as you walk to the stage, imagine the audience in rapturous applause, delighted to see you and eager to hear what you have to say.

▲ Imagine your audience in their underwear

If you have a really tough time with nerves, try and imagine your audience in a ridiculous situation like sitting on the toilet or in their underwear.

33

Dealing with disaster

If you are well prepared, your presentation will usually go well, but some things are beyond your control. Here are some ideas on how to cope when things go wrong.

▲ The computer fails

No matter how well prepared you are, sometimes technology fails. If you are at a big meeting there will probably be some technical assistance, so provided you have a backup copy of your slides on floppy disc or CD you can continue with a replacement machine. Otherwise, it may be a good idea to take a backup copy of your presentation on OHP slides. In teaching situations, if you have provided hard copy of all your slides as a handout, you can take your audience through the presentation slide-by-slide.

▲ The previous speaker covers things you wanted to say

In this situation you really have to think on your feet. One technique is to refer back to the previous speaker, acknowledge what they said, and give more detail than you had originally planned on your own work.

▲ Someone comes up with a devastating question

When someone poses a question to which you have no answer, you can sometimes buy time by reflecting it back to the audience with 'Does anyone here have any experience in this area?' or 'I would just like to get a feel for what the audience thinks about this point'. Sometimes, there may be an eminent authority in the room to whom you can refer: 'It would be remiss of me to comment before asking Professor Smith's view, as this is her field'. If you are really stuck, it's better to admit you don't know than to bluster and risk losing credibility. With student questions, you can offer to research the answer and get back to them at the next session – or ask them to research the answer themselves.

▲ You forget what you're going to say

Even experienced presenters can lose track of their presentations. If – or rather when – this happens, the main priority is to stay calm and not to panic. Pausing to look at your notes will often get things going again and it will appear to be very natural to the audience. Alternatively, in a teaching situation, you can turn to someone in the audience and ask them to recap on the main points or ask them a question while you gather your thoughts together.

▲ You freeze

What if panic sets in and you find yourself rooted to the spot with a completely blank mind? Take a few deep breaths, and smile at a friendly face in the audience. In extreme cases, carry a sharp object like a key in your pocket and grip it firmly. The sensation of physical pain stops you from thinking of anything else while you refer to your notes. To prevent the build-up of panic before you rise to speak, occupy your mind with some displacement activity such as counting backwards from 600 in fives.

34

Answering questions

The way in which you handle questions is an important part of the total presentation. It can be daunting, but is also a good opportunity to demonstrate your knowledge of your subject and exchange information with others.

▲ Be clear about when questions will be taken

At larger conferences, the meeting organisers will often make an announcement about whether questions will be taken at the end of each presentation, or whether there will be a panel discussion after several presentations. In less formal situations, you should decide about whether you will take questions during the presentation or wait until the end. Generally speaking, questions of clarification can be handled during the presentation, whereas others should be left to the end to avoid disturbing the flow.

▲ Treat a question as a compliment

Try and treat a question as a compliment and not a challenge – it shows that someone was interested enough to think of a question.

▲ Imagine possible questions and prepare for them

Think carefully beforehand about what the likely questions will be and plan your responses. Try your presentation out on some friendly colleagues who can suggest possible questions, including the difficult-to-answer ones.

▲ Listen carefully to the question

Make sure you listen carefully to the whole question. Do not be afraid to ask for clarification.

▲ If it is impossible to understand the question, postpone answering

Occasionally, if there is a language barrier between you and the questioner, it may be impossible to understand the question in the time available. At this point, the chairperson should ideally intervene, but if they do not, say 'I'm very sorry, I'm having some trouble understanding the question, but I'd like to answer you. Would you mind if we talked at the coffee break?'

▲ Repeat the question before you answer it

Repeating the question before you answer it will buy valuable thinking time and will also make sure that the whole audience has heard and understood the question.

▲ Don't patronise the questioner

Try to avoid saying 'That's a good question' – it can sound patronising.

▲ Keep your answers short and to the point

Keep your answers short, simple and relevant. This will allow time for more questions.

▲ Look at the questioner and act confidently

Give the questioner two-thirds of your eye contact whilst responding. Watch your body language and try to control any tell-tale signs of unease.

▲ Don't waste time if you will be covering the point later

If someone asks a question that will be covered later on, say so and move on to the next question.

▲ Be positive and friendly, even if your questioner is not

Always respond positively, even if the questioner is being negative. Back away rather than allow yourself to be drawn into an argument. The chairperson should intervene if a discussion is turning into a row. Alternatively, you can simply say 'I think this is too big a question to resolve in a few minutes. Let's have the next question, and we can talk separately about these issues later.'

35

Handling difficult people in seminar groups

Generally, your audience wants you to succeed. However, in small-group teaching situations you can occasionally come up against difficult people or situations that need skilful handling.

▲ Acknowledge dominant people, but don't allow them to railroad the seminar

Some people have a natural urge to dominate in any situation. However, as the presenter, you want to maintain control over the flow of material and the direction the seminar is taking. Avoid seeing this as a battle in which the dominant person must be silenced. Instead, balance their contribution, making sure that they are heard but that they do not constantly interrupt.

▲ Be firm with unreasonable interruptions

If the same point is being made continually, say 'I understand your point, and it's unfortunate that today we don't have the time to debate it fully'.

▲ Avoid prolonged eye contact with the dominant person

Rather like an angry dog, a dominant person can perceive sustained eye contact as a challenge.

▲ Be neutral if seminar participants argue

Even if you would naturally side with one participant rather than another, stay neutral. Try to slow the conflict down, allowing one person to speak at a time and disallowing rude interruptions. Answer any direct questions in a direct and honest way, and try to avoid feeling personally affronted.

▲ Try not to get drawn into the emotions of others

Keep calm and remember that conflict is not necessarily bad. Recognise that people tend to be more assertive or even aggressive when an issue is important to them.

▲ Listen before you try to intervene in a heated discussion

Listen to what is being said. Are the positions really opposed, or is there a misunderstanding that you can clarify to both participants?

▲ Don't try to stop a row too abruptly

Pushing the conflict to one side will create frustration and cause it to blow up again later. If you need to, suggest a private meeting to debate the issues further.

▲ Try to make sure everyone has the chance to be involved

Watch the seminar group and look for anyone who is not participating. This could be because they have nothing to say, but may also be because they feel too shy to speak or are intimidated by more vocal members of the group.

▲ Give less assertive people the chance to speak ...

You can try asking questions whilst looking at the person – open questions about opinions rather than facts will help to avoid embarrassing them if they have no answer. If everyone in the group is quiet, you can also try leaving long pauses after questions to try to encourage someone else to step in and fill the silence. However, this can be rather stressful if no one says anything!

▲ ... But do not force people to take part

Recognise that not every person is able or wishes to fully participate in an open meeting, so do not persist in trying to get them to speak when others are perfectly happy to do so.

▲ Keep control by curbing the 'ramblers'

If someone keeps on talking long after they have made their point, do not be afraid to interrupt, but pick your moment carefully. If you wait until the speaker changes tack slightly, the interruption is less obvious and avoids embarrassing them.

▲ When you do interrupt a 'rambler', acknowledge the value of their contribution

Summarise any valuable information briefly, and appeal to their sense of 'fair play' by saying that specific others wish to add their comments.

▲ Keep your ears open for distracting side conversations

There are three possible approaches:

- Move physically into the group near the 'talkers' but don't look directly at them (this is too obvious).
- Use silence, so that they suddenly find that everyone can hear them.
- Address them directly by saying 'I can hear some good points being made, I wonder if we could address some of these issues as a group?' But don't do this to deliberately humiliate them if they weren't actually discussing the topic.

▲ Look out for participants with confused expressions

Address their body language directly, taking responsibility: 'I may not have made that last point as clear as I might. What I meant was …' Then recap on the points made and check understanding. You can also ask members of the audience to summarise what's just been said, covertly helping those who didn't get it the first time round.

▲ Note that a confused expression may indicate poor eyesight

If someone is wrinkling their brow and screwing up their eyes, it may not indicate that they are confused by what you've just said – they may simply be trying to make out what's on the screen. Say to the audience 'If any of you can't see the screen very well, please move down to the front' – that way you won't embarrass one individual.

▲ Be prepared to encounter negative reactions occasionally

If someone appears excessively negative or antagonistic, try not to take it personally. There will be a valid reason for the feeling (which may be quite unrelated to you or the topic of the seminar). Try to bring out and handle any factual objections they may have to your presentation, and show willingness to listen and debate. Sometimes, however, there may be no factual issues that you can address. In that case, it's not your job to try to make them happy – just leave them to their feelings and work with the rest of the group.

▲ Remember that most people want you to succeed

Even if you do encounter difficult people from time to time, the group as a whole is likely to want you to succeed. Often other members of the group will step in and deal with difficult people before you have to tackle them yourself.

Index